STUDENT WORKBOOK TO ACCOMPANY

NURSING ASSISTANT

Basics

Barbara R. Hegner, MSN, RN
(deceased)

Barbara Acello, MS, RN
Independent Nurse Consultant and Educator

Esther Caldwell

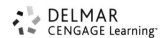

DELMAR
CENGAGE Learning

Australia • Brazil • Japan • Korea • Mexico • Singapore • Spain • United Kingdom • United States

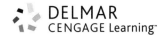
DELMAR
CENGAGE Learning™

**Workbook to Accompany Nursing Assistant:
A Nursing Process Approach—BASICS**
Barbara R. Hegner, Barbara Acello,
and Esther Caldwell

Vice President, Career and Professional
Editorial: Dave Garza

Director of Learning Solutions: Matthew Kane

Senior Acquisitions Editor: Maureen Rosener

Managing Editor: Marah Bellegarde

Product Manager: Jadin Babin-Kavanaugh

Editorial Assistant: Samantha Miller

Vice President, Career and Professional
Marketing: Jennifer McAvey

Executive Marketing Manager: Michele McTighe

Marketing Coordinator: Scott Chrysler

Production Director: Carolyn Miller

Production Manager: Andrew Crouth

Senior Content Project Manager:
Kenneth McGrath

Senior Art Director: Jack Pendleton

For product information and technology assistance, contact us at
Cengage Learning Customer & Sales Support, 1-800-354-9706

For permission to use material from this text or product,
submit all requests online at **www.cengage.com/permissions**
Further permissions questions can be emailed to
permissionrequest@cengage.com

Library of Congress Control Number: 2009925904

ISBN-13: 978-1-4283-1747-5

ISBN-10: 1-4283-1747-3

Delmar
Executive Woods
5 Maxwell Drive
Clifton Park, NY 12065
USA

Cengage Learning is a leading provider of customized learning solutions with office locations around the globe, including Singapore, the United Kingdom, Australia, Mexico, Brazil, and Japan. Locate your local office at **www.cengage.com/global**

Cengage Learning products are represented in Canada by Nelson Education, Ltd.

To learn more about Delmar, visit **www.cengage.com/delmar**

Purchase any of our products at your local bookstore or at our preferred online store **www.cengagebrain.com**

Notice to the Reader

Publisher does not warrant or guarantee any of the products described herein or perform any independent analysis in connection with any of the product information contained herein. Publisher does not assume, and expressly disclaims, any obligation to obtain and include information other than that provided to it by the manufacturer. The reader is expressly warned to consider and adopt all safety precautions that might be indicated by the activities described herein and to avoid all potential hazards. By following the instructions contained herein, the reader willingly assumes all risks in connection with such instructions. The publisher makes no representations or warranties of any kind, including but not limited to, the warranties of fitness for particular purpose or merchantability, nor are any such representations implied with respect to the material set forth herein, and the publisher takes no responsibility with respect to such material. The publisher shall not be liable for any special, consequential, or exemplary damages resulting, in whole or part, from the readers' use of, or reliance upon, this material.

Printed in the United States of America
2 3 4 5 6 7 16 15 14 13 12

CONTENTS

TO THE LEARNER

The content of this workbook follows a basic organizational plan. Each lesson in the workbook includes:

- Behavioral objectives.
- A summary of the related unit in the *Nursing Assistant Basics* text.
- Exercises to help you review, recall, and reinforce concepts that have been taught.
- Nursing Assistant Alerts, which are key points to remember about each unit. The Alerts are reminders of the important concepts of the unit and the benefits to be obtained from them.
- Opportunities to apply nursing assistant care to the nursing process and expand your horizons.

It has been shown that students who complete a special guide as they learn new materials perform better, have greater confidence, and are more secure in the basic concepts than those who do not.

You may wish to complete the workbook activities in preparation for your class, or after class, while the information is fresh in your mind. In either case, the workbook and classwork will reinforce each other.

You can make the best use of the workbook if you:

- Read and study the related chapter in the text.
- Observe and listen carefully to your instructor's explanations and demonstrations.
- Read over the behavioral objectives before you start the workbook and then check to be sure you have met them after you complete the lesson exercises.
- Use the summary to review the chapter content.
- Complete the activities in the workbook. Circle any questions you are unable to finish to discuss with your instructor at the next class meeting.

It is the authors' sincere desire that the workbook will offer you support as you learn to become the best possible nursing assistant.

You have chosen a special goal for yourself. You have decided to become a knowledgeable, skilled nursing assistant. Keep this goal in mind, but realize that to reach it, you need to take many small steps. Each step you master takes you closer to your ultimate goal.

Barbara Acello

THE LEARNING PROCESS

Students may feel anxious about the learning process. However, learning really can be pleasurable and rewarding if you have an open mind, a desire to succeed, and a willingness to follow some simple steps.

You have already won half the battle, because you have entered an educational program. This shows your desire to accomplish a real-life goal: to become a nursing assistant.

There are three basic steps to learning:

1. Active listening

2. Effective studying

3. Careful practicing

Active Listening

Listening actively is not easy, natural, or passive. It is, however, a skill that can be learned. Good listeners are not born, they are made. Studies show that the average listening efficiency in this culture is only about 25%. That means that although you may *hear* (a passive action) all that is said, you actually listen to and process only about one-quarter of the material. Effective listening requires a conscious effort by the listener. The most neglected communication skill is listening.

An important part of your work as a nursing assistant involves active listening to patients and coworkers. To learn this skill properly, you must begin to listen actively to your instructor or supervisor. Hearing but not processing information puts you and your patient in jeopardy.

Active listening is listening with personal involvement. There are three actions in active listening:

- Hearing what is said (passive action)

- Processing the information (active action)

- Using the information (active action)

Hearing What Is Said

People speak at an average rate of 125 words per minute. You must pay close attention to the speaker to hear what is said. This is not difficult if you do not let other thoughts and sounds interfere with your thinking. If you sit up straight and lean forward in the classroom or stand erect in the clinical area, your whole body is more receptive. Position yourself where you can adequately see or hear and keep your attention focused on the speaker. Make eye contact if possible and remain alert.

Many distractions can break your concentration unless you take action to prevent them from doing so. For example, distractions may be:

- Interruptions, such as other activities in the classroom or in the patient's unit that catch your attention or create noise.

- Daydreaming and thinking about personal activities or problems.

- Physical fatigue. Adequate sleep and rest are powerful aids to the ability to concentrate.

- Lack of interest, because you cannot immediately see the importance of the information.

To be an effective listener, you must actively work at eliminating these distractions. You must put energy into staying focused.

Processing the Information

Remember that hearing the words is not enough. You must actively *process* (make sense of) the words in your brain. You must put meaning to them, and that takes effort. There are things you can do to improve the process. These include:

- Interact with the speaker using eye contact, smiles, and nods.

- Ask meaningful questions. Contribute your own comments if it is a discussion.

- Take notes.

These actions allow your memory to establish relationships with previously learned knowledge and to make new connections.

Taking notes gives you another way to imprint what you are processing. You are not only hearing the sounds of the words, but also seeing the important words on paper. Note-taking helps you recall points that you may have forgotten.

Note-taking is a skill that can be learned. If used, it will greatly improve the learning process. You may need to take notes in class, during demonstrations, and when your supervisor or instructor gives you a clinical assignment. Here are some hints to make developing this skill easier:

- Come prepared with a pencil and paper.

- Don't try to write down every word.

- Write down only the important points or key words.

- Learn to take notes in an outline form.

- Listen with particular care to the beginning sentence. It usually reveals the primary purpose.

- Pay special attention to the final statement. It is often a summary.

Outlines include the important points summarized in a meaningful way. Be sure to leave room so that you can add material.

There are different ways of outlining. One way is to use letters and numbers to designate important points. Another is to draw a pattern of lines to show relationships. Use either way or one of your own design, but be consistent. Practice helps you master the skill of outlining.

As you make notes of material that is not clear, add a star or some other mark next to the material. When the speaker asks for questions, you can quickly find yours.

If the speaker stresses a point, be sure to mark your outline by underlining the information. This will call special attention to these points when you use the outline for study.

After class, you can reorganize your notes and compare them to your text readings.

Effective Studying

Here are some general tips to help you study better.

- Feel certain that each lesson you master is important to prepare your knowledge and skills. The workbook, text, and instructor materials have been carefully coordinated to meet the objectives. Review the objectives before you begin to study. They are like a road map that will take you to your goal.

- Remember that you are the learner, so you can take credit for your success. The instructor is an important guide and the workbook, text, and clinical experiences are tools, but you are the learner and whether you use the tools wisely is finally up to you.

- Take an honest look at yourself and your study habits. Take positive steps to avoid habits that could limit your success. For example, do you let family responsibilities or social opportunities interfere with study times? If so, sit down with your family and plan a schedule for study that they will support and to which you will adhere. Find a special place to study that is free from distraction. If the telephone interferes, take it off the hook or let everyone know that this is your study time.

The Study Plan

Plan a schedule for study. Actually sit down and write out a weekly schedule, hour by hour, so that you know exactly how your time is being spent. Then plan specific study time, but be realistic. Study has to be balanced with the other activities of your life. Learn to budget your time so that you have time to prepare and study on a regular basis and block in extra time when tests are scheduled. Don't forget to block in time for fun as well! Look back over the week to see how well you have kept to your schedule. If you had difficulty, try to adjust the schedule to better meet your needs. If you were successful, pat yourself on the back. You have done very well!

Make your study area special. It need not be elaborate, but make sure there is ample light. You should have a desk to work on and a supply of paper and pencils. Sharpen your pencils at the end of each study period and leave papers readily at hand. You may think this sounds strange, but people often waste time at the beginning of a study session with these mechanical tasks. If these things are ready when you first sit down, you can get started without distractions or delay. Keep your medical dictionary in your work area. When you get home, put your text and workbook there also. In other words, your work area should be designed for study. When you treat it this way, you will find that as soon as you sit down there, you will be psychologically prepared to study.

Class Study

Now that you have your study area and work schedule organized, you need to think about how you can get the most out of your class experience.

- First, come prepared. Read the behavioral objectives and the lesson before class. This prepares you by acquainting you with the focus of the lesson and the vocabulary.

- Listen actively as the instructor explains the lesson. Keep your mind on what the instructor is saying. If your thoughts start to wander, refocus immediately.

- Take notes on the special points that are stressed. Use these as you study at home.

- Participate in class discussions. Remember that discussion subjects are chosen because they relate to the lesson. You can learn much from hearing the comments of others and by contributing your own. Pay attention to slides, films, and overhead transparencies, because these offer a visual approach to the subject matter. You might even take notes on important points during a film or jot down questions you would like the instructor to answer.

- Ask intelligent and pertinent questions. Make sure your questions are simple and centered on the topic. Focus on one point at a time and write down the answers for later review.

- Use any models and charts that are available. Study them and see how they apply to the lesson.

- Carefully observe the demonstrations your instructor gives. Note in your book any change that may have been made in the procedure steps to conform with the policy of your facility or state.

- Perform return demonstrations carefully in the classroom. Remember, you are learning skills that will be used with real patients in the clinical situation.

After Class

When class is over and you have had a break, you are ready to settle down and study. You can gain the most from the experience by:

- Studying in your prepared study area. Everything will be ready and waiting for you if you followed the first part of this plan.

- Read over the lesson, beginning with the behavioral objectives.

- Read with a highlighter or pencil in hand so you can underline or highlight important material.

- Answer the questions at the end of the unit. Check any you found difficult by reviewing that section of the text.

- Complete the related workbook unit.

- Review the behavioral objectives at the beginning of the unit. Ask yourself if you have met them. If not, go back and review. Prepare the next day's lesson by reading over the next day's unit.

- Use the medical dictionary for words you may learn that are not in the text glossary. The dictionary provides pronunciations.

Study Groups

Studying with someone else who is trying to learn the same material can be very helpful and supportive, but there are some pitfalls you must avoid. If studying with someone else is to be effective and productive:

- Limit the number of people studying to a maximum of three; one other person is best.

- Keep focused on the subject. Don't begin to talk about classmates or the day's social events.

- Come prepared for the study session. Have your work completed. Use the study session to reinforce your learning and explore deeper understanding of the material.

- Ask each other questions about the materials.

- Make a list of things to ask your instructor.

- Limit the study session to a specific length. Follow the plan and you will succeed!

OBJECTIVES

After completing this unit, you will be able to:

- Spell and define terms.
- Describe the effect of study skills on successful learning.
- Write the steps involved in active listening.
- List things that interfere with effective listening.
- Use two techniques of note-taking.
- Name ways to improve study habits.
- Effectively use the textbook.

UNIT SUMMARY

Developing effective study habits can be important to a lifetime of learning. A few simple steps can make the process easier.

- Become familiar with your text. It will save time in locating information.
- Practice the steps to learning by being an active listener.
- Take notes for reference and study.
- Plan study times and practice in ways that promote learning.

ACTIVITIES

Vocabulary Exercise

Define the words in the spaces provided.

1. active listening

_____

2. end-of-unit materials

_____

3. processing

_____

4. behavioral objectives

_____

5. glossary

_____

Completion

Complete the statements in the spaces provided.

1. Behavioral objectives help to direct your _____

2. There are three basic steps to learning: _____, _____,

   and _____.

3. Daydreaming can _____ with your ability to listen actively.

4. Planning a schedule of classes and other responsibilities will help you use study time more

   _____.

5. Use the _____ to learn the meaning of new terms and words.

6. Follow the maze. Which path will you travel?

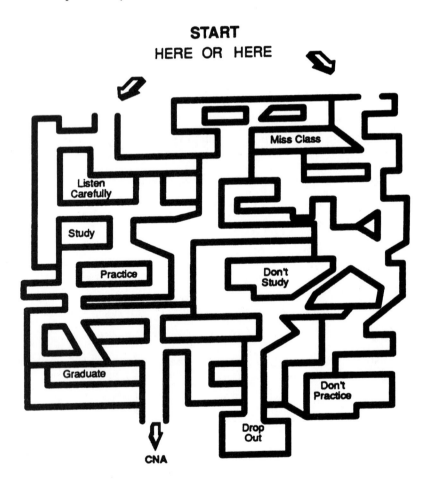

7. Name techniques of note-taking.

   a. _____

   b. _____

8. Read the following case history. Then use one of the two note-taking techniques to outline the material.

Victoria Bohn was 8½ months pregnant when she first appeared at our family planning clinic. The mother of three lively little girls, ages 13 months, 2 years, and 3 years, she looked tired as her children pulled at her skirt and fussed.

When her turn came to be examined, the nursing assistant found that her blood pressure was 148/100, pulse 92, respiration 24, temperature 103°F. Her hands and fingers were swollen, and she complained of pain in her abdomen high on the right side. She had gained 38 pounds since becoming pregnant. Concerned, the nursing assistant informed the nurse.

After examining Ms. Bohn and listening to her baby's heartbeat, Mrs. Edelson, the registered nurse supervising the clinic, told Ms. Bohn that she wanted the physician to examine her. When the physician made his examination, he immediately recommended that Ms. Bohn be admitted to the acute care hospital.

During her hospitalization, it was found that the patient had a severe infection in her abdomen, which was successfully treated with antibiotics. While in the hospital, her blood pressure and fluid levels were brought within normal limits.

Ms. Bohn remained in the hospital until delivery of a beautiful 8-pound girl. A grandmother, who had been helping take care of the family, agreed to remain in the home for a period of time until Ms. Bohn was once again able to manage her family herself.

_____

_____

_____

_____

_____

_____

_____

_____

_____

_____

_____

_____

_____

_____

_____

_____

_____

_____

Student Activities

Introduction to Nursing Assisting

Community Health Care

OBJECTIVES

After completing this unit, you will be able to:

- Spell and define terms.
- List the five basic functions of health care facilities.
- Describe the differences between acute care and long-term care.
- Name at least five departments within a hospital and state their functions.
- Describe patient-focused care.
- State the purpose of health care facility surveys.

UNIT SUMMARY

- Health care facilities provide health care to members of the community.

- Specific care is provided in different types of facilities.

- Nursing assistants play an important role in this caregiving.

- Many changes have occurred within the past few years, brought about by increased aging of the general population, new technologies, and the need to contain costs.

- Different workers work as a team in various departments to meet the community's health needs.

- Health care facilities must comply with health and safety laws and regulations, and undertake activities to ensure quality.

ACTIVITIES

Vocabulary Exercise

Define the words in the spaces provided.

1. facility

_____

2. hospice

_____

3. patient

_____

4. pediatric

_____

5. community

_____

Completion

Complete the statements in the spaces provided.

1. List five basic functions of all health care facilities.

    a. _____

    b. _____

    c. _____

    d. _____

    e. _____

2. Patient-focused care means

_____

3. The cost of health care has increased because of demand for services as a result of

_____

4. The person receiving care in an acute care hospital is called a

_____

5. Give three examples of health care facilities.

    a. _____

    b. _____

    c. _____

6. Three names applied to the person receiving care are

    a. _____

    b. _____

    c. _____

7. A health care facility survey is done to

_____

8. The Occupational Safety and Health Administration is a governmental agency that

_____

Word Search

Find the following words in the puzzle and put a circle around each word. Define each word in the spaces provided.

r	j	j	n	u	c	i	n	o	r	h	c	s	i
p	e	n	e	q	k	o	u	t	u	g	u	h	m
r	k	h	p	u	b	b	u	y	k	r	w	o	m
e	b	m	a	m	c	t	d	m	v	l	m	s	u
n	z	a	f	b	h	h	n	e	m	u	g	p	z
a	t	p	a	e	i	a	y	u	s	z	o	i	n
t	n	x	p	v	m	l	t	u	d	x	d	c	o
a	v	h	b	k	a	r	i	g	b	k	x	e	i
l	g	e	w	w	a	u	k	t	z	m	q	n	t
e	g	u	p	p	z	n	v	z	a	t	u	u	a
j	a	m	t	t	x	c	w	k	w	t	h	o	t
h	v	s	z	k	q	l	p	x	y	q	i	q	i
z	o	p	a	t	i	e	n	t	w	k	w	o	c
p	r	m	m	c	y	t	i	l	i	c	a	f	n

1. hospice

_____

2. postpartum

_____

3. prenatal

_____

4. facility

_____

5. survey

_____

6. rehabilitation

_____

7. citation

_____

8. chronic

_____

9. patient

_____

DEVELOPING GREATER INSIGHT

1. Chad is thinking of studying to be a nursing assistant. He tells you he has heard the term *patient-focused care*, and asks you what it means. Explain this term to him using words he will understand.

_____

_____

_____

_____

2. After you define *patient-focused care* for him, Chad asks you how this type of care affects nursing assistant practice. What will you tell him?

_____

_____

_____

_____

3. You have just taken a job at the county hospital close to your home. A former classmate calls you and informs you that she was hired at the teaching hospital associated with the state university. She says to call her if you have any questions about policies and procedures. Is this a good idea? Why or why not?

_____

_____

_____

_____

On the Job: Being a Nursing Assistant

OBJECTIVES

After completing this unit, you will be able to:

- Spell and define terms.
- Identify the members of the interdisciplinary health care team.
- Identify the members of the nursing team.
- Understand the legal limits of nursing assistant practice.
- List the job responsibilities of the nursing assistant.
- State the purpose of evidence-based practice.
- Make a chart showing your facility's lines of authority.
- Discuss the potential for career growth and advancement.
- Describe the importance of good human relationships and list ways of building productive relationships with patients, families, and staff.
- List the rules of personal hygiene and explain the importance of a healthy mental attitude.
- Describe the appropriate dress for the job.

UNIT SUMMARY

- Nursing practice is evidence-based. This means that procedures are identified and decisions made based on the strength of the evidence, which is research-based.

- A nursing assessment is the basis for nursing care. Nursing assistants contribute data and information to the total assessment.

- *Delegation* is the transfer of responsibility for the performance of a nursing activity from a nurse to someone who does not already have the authority. The nurse practice act serves as a guide for delegation.

- Delegation is not appropriate in all situations. For successful delegation, the right task must be delegated to the right person in the right circumstances. Communication must be accurate and supervision adequate.

- Hand-off communication must be accurate, clear, and complete, and must provide an opportunity to ask questions.

Nursing assistants:

- Have specific responsibilities that vary within different agencies, but must always function within the scope of nursing assistant practice.

- Must follow established procedures and policies.

- Represent themselves and their agency or facility. Good grooming is essential.

- Are ultimately responsible for their own actions.

- Must develop good interpersonal relationships with patients, visitors, and coworkers. This helps nursing assistants to be more effective.

- Will find that personal adjustments are made easier by understanding and obeying facility policies and procedures.

- Must always treat patients, coworkers, and visitors with dignity.

- Must take a written or oral and clinical test to become certified.

- May be cross-trained to increase their skills.

- Must be well organized and have good time management skills.

- Should establish and develop a systematic daily routine for making rounds and planning care as assigned.

NURSING ASSISTANT ALERT

Action	Benefit
Maintain good grooming.	Enhances appearance and health. Inspires patient confidence.
Make sure uniform is complete.	Identifies your role and responsibilities.
Practice stress reduction.	Keeps you mentally and emotionally stable.

ACTIVITIES

Vocabulary Exercise

Define the words in the spaces provided.

1. attitude

_____

2. burnout

_____

3. nursing team

_____

4. scope of practice

_____

5. nursing assistant

_____

6. hand-off communication

_____

Completion

Complete the statements in the spaces provided.

1. Write four terms used to identify the nursing assistant.

   a. _____

   b. _____

   c. _____

   d. _____

2. List three members of the nursing team.

   a. _____

   b. _____

   c. _____

3. Explain what is meant by the "line of authority."

   _____

4. What should you do if you have any doubts about your assignment?

   _____

5. Name three characteristics of a successful nursing assistant.

   a. _____

   b. _____

   c. _____

6. List three activities you could carry out to ensure good personal hygiene.

   a. _____

   b. _____

   c. _____

7. Explain why wearing jewelry is unwise when you are on duty.

   _____

8. What jewelry is part of your uniform?

   _____

9. The main concern of every nursing assistant should be the well-being and

   _____

10. List four reasons why a patient might be irritable, complaining, or uncooperative.

    a. _____

    b. _____

    c. _____

    d. _____

11. List three dimensions in which patients have needs.

    a. _____

    b. _____

    c. _____

12. List five ways you can ensure good working relationships.

a. _____

b. _____

c. _____

d. _____

e. _____

13. For each of the following grooming traits, check whether the trait is a positive or a negative trait in a nursing assistant.

Trait	Positive	Negative
a. long hair		
b. clean shoelaces		
c. cigarette odor		
d. bright nail polish		
e. unpolished shoes		
f. dangling earrings		
g. light lipstick		
h. long fingernails		
i. use of antiperspirant/deodorant		

14. Explain why stress is an issue for all nursing assistants and how you can reduce its effects.

_____

15. Complete the chart to demonstrate the proper lines of communication.

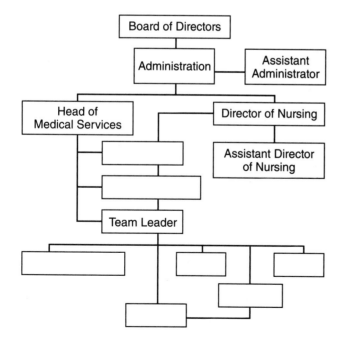

Matching

Match the specialist and the type of care provided.

Type of Care

Specialist

1. _____ Cares for the aging person
2. _____ Treats and diagnoses disorders of the eye
3. _____ Treats disorders of the skin
4. _____ Treats disorders of the digestive system
5. _____ Treats disorders of the heart and blood vessels
6. _____ Treats and diagnoses disorders of the nervous system
7. _____ Treats disorders of the blood
8. _____ Cares for women during pregnancy
9. _____ Diagnoses and treats with X-rays
10. _____ Treats disorders of the mind

a. Cardiologist

b. Gastroenterologist

c. Neurologist

d. Radiologist

e. Obstetrician

f. Hematologist

g. Psychiatrist

h. Ophthalmologist

i. Gerontologist

j. Dermatologist

DEVELOPING GREATER INSIGHT

1. The nurse asks you to help her get Mrs. Scornavacco's assessment done so she can work on the care plan before the family members arrive for a scheduled care plan meeting. She asks you to obtain the patient's weight using the bed scale, measure her height, and take the vital signs. Your instructor emphasized that nursing assistants are not permitted to complete assessments. How will you handle this situation?

_____

_____

_____

_____

2. Mary, another nursing assistant, calls you aside. She is very upset. She thinks the nurse is mad at her because Mary was assigned to take Mr. Turnbull's 8:00 PM vital signs. Mr. Turnbull is unstable, and the doctor is considering a transfer to the critical care unit. When Mary arrived in the room at 7:51 PM, the nurse had just finished taking the vital signs. The nurse seemed rushed and left the room without saying a word about the vital signs or Mary's assignment. What will you tell Mary? Why?

_____

_____

_____

_____

Consumer Rights and Responsibilities in Health Care

UNIT SUMMARY

Consumer rights protect patients and ensure optimum care. They are spelled out in special documents such as the:

- Patients' Bill of Rights

- Clients' Rights in Home Care

- Residents' Rights

Consumer rights are protected and optimal care is better ensured when consumers participate in the process by:

- Sharing health histories openly

- Participating in their own care to the extent possible

- Accepting financial responsibility

- Being sure they understand care directions

- Living a healthful lifestyle

NURSING ASSISTANT ALERT

Action	Benefit
Understand and be guided by consumer rights	Protects patients. Ensures optimal care.

ACTIVITIES

Vocabulary Exercise

Using the definitions, unscramble the words in the puzzle that identify documents designed to protect consumers of health care.

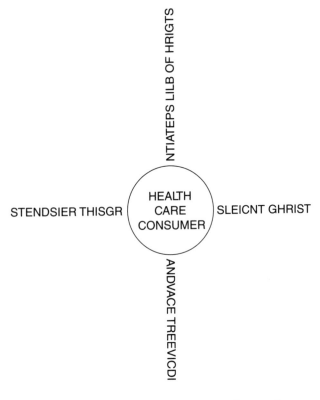

1. Given to patients upon admission to a hospital

_____

2. Relates to people receiving care at home

_____

3. Given to people before admission to a long-term care facility

_____

4. Gives instructions about consumers' wishes regarding care when they are unable to make their wishes known

_____

Completion

Complete the following statements by using the correct term(s) from the list provided. Some may be used more than once.

accept	clarification	Clients' Rights	federal
financial	honestly	medications	past
Patients' Bill of Rights	responsibility	will not	

1. The Omnibus Budget Reconciliation Act of 1987 is _____ legislation.

2. A copy of the _____ is given to a person upon admission to a hospital.

3. A copy of the _____ is given to consumers during the first home visit.

4. Consumers have a _____ to maintain personal health care records.

5. Consumers are responsible for communicating _____ with the physician and other caregivers.

6. It is important for consumers to provide accurate information regarding _____ hospitalizations and _____.

7. Consumers are responsible for informing health care providers if they _____ be able to carry out prescribed treatment.

8. Consumers must _____ responsibility for learning how to manage their own health.

9. Consumers are responsible for asking for _____ if they do not fully understand instructions.

10. Consumers must assume _____ responsibility for health care.

True/False

Mark the following true or false by circling T or F.

1. T F All citizens in the United States have certain rights that are guaranteed by law.

2. T F Consumers have no rights once they enter a health care facility.

3. T F The Omnibus Budget Reconciliation Act of 1987 was enacted by the federal government to ensure the rights of patients in acute care facilities.

4. T F *Informed consent* means that the person gives permission for care even if he or she does not fully understand the purpose of the care.

5. T F A grievance is a situation in which the consumer feels there are grounds for a complaint.

6. T F Both caregiver and consumer have responsibilities that help ensure optimal health care.

7. T F Patients have the right to determine the cost of care.

8. T F All personal and clinical records pertaining to a patient must be kept confidential.

9. T F Unless a consumer gives consent, an experimental procedure may not be performed.

10. T F In long-term care, visitors may be restricted against the resident's wishes.

11. T F Patients have a role in making treatment choices and planning care.

12. T F Patients have the right to open and honest communication with caregivers.

13. T F A patient who feels that he has been injured must keep this information to himself.

14. T F A resident has the right to choose an attending physician.

15. T F The resident has the right to freedom from corporal punishment.

16. T   F   Patients must accept the treatment prescribed by their physicians.

17. T   F   Patients do not have the right to examine their medical bills as long as the insurance company is paying those bills.

18. T   F   Patients have the right to know if the physician and other health workers are in business together.

Identification

Determine the appropriateness of a nursing assistant's behavior by indicating C for correct or I for incorrect.

1. _____ Listening to visitors' conversations.

2. _____ Discussing a patient's physical status with one of the patient's relatives.

3. _____ Making shift reports so that patients cannot hear.

4. _____ Reading a patient's record to satisfy your curiosity.

5. _____ Sharing the medical records with the patient's minister.

6. _____ Telling a patient that her roommate has a terminal condition.

7. _____ Telling another nursing assistant that a patient eats best when fed from the right side.

8. _____ Informing another staff member that the patient is incontinent.

9. _____ Telling another patient that a roommate has dirty toenails.

10. _____ Mentioning that a patient has beautiful white hair to the patient's roommate.

11. _____ Treating patients with dignity and respect.

12. _____ Handling a patient's personal items carefully.

13. _____ Not telling the client your name before beginning care.

14. _____ Letting a client know that someone else will be making the next visit.

15. _____ Not allowing the client to assist with a bath when he is able to do so.

16. _____ Explaining restrictions on the number of visitors each patient may have while in intensive care.

17. _____ Referring the patient's question about his blood pressure to the nurse.

18. _____ Telling the patient's daughter that her father does not have long to live.

DEVELOPING GREATER INSIGHT

1. Susan Lupine is a patient on your unit. Your neighbor tells you that Susan "has AIDS," and asks you if her sudden admission to the hospital is due to a complication of AIDS. You are not aware that Susan has been diagnosed with HIV or AIDS. She was admitted to your unit after an emergency appendectomy. She is receiving IV antibiotics because her appendix ruptured prior to surgery. Will you tell your neighbor that Susan had emergency surgery? Why or why not? Will you address the rumor about HIV/AIDS with the neighbor or at work? Why or why not?

_____

_____

_____

_____

Ethical and Legal Issues Affecting the Nursing Assistant

OBJECTIVES

After completing this unit, you will be able to:

- Spell and define terms.
- Describe the legal responsibilities of a nursing assistant.
- Describe how to protect patients' right to privacy.
- Define abuse and neglect, and give examples of each.
- Define sexual harassment and give examples of activities that may be perceived as being sexually harassing.

UNIT SUMMARY

All persons giving health care voluntarily adhere to a set of ethical standards. They agree to:

- Protect life
- Promote health
- Keep personal information confidential
- Respect personal beliefs about death
- Give care based on need, not gratuities (tips)
- Provide safety

Nursing assistants have legal responsibilities. Legal situations the health care provider wants to avoid include:

- Negligence
- Assault and battery
- Theft
- Invasion of privacy
- Abuse
- Malpractice
- Neglect

NURSING ASSISTANT ALERT

Action	Benefit
Maintain ethical standards.	Protects patients' rights and privacy.
Obey laws.	Protects you against legal actions and keeps patient safe.
Carry out orders or report inability to do so to supervisor.	Ensures proper and safe nursing care.
Protect patients' physical and personal privacy.	Makes patients feel secure and protected.

ACTIVITIES

Vocabulary Exercise

Define the words in the spaces provided.

1. confidential

_____

2. assault

_____

3. negligence

_____

4. verbal abuse

_____

5. slander

_____

6. malpractice

_____

7. neglect

_____

Completion

Complete the statements in the spaces provided.

1. Ethical standards are a _____ code rather than a legal code.

2. State the purpose of the ethics committee.

_____

_____

_____

_____

3. List five ways to ensure that the patient receives the proper treatment.

a. _____

b. _____

c. _____

d. _____

e. _____

4. The patient offers you a tip for getting him fresh water. Describe and explain your response.

_____

5. You have not stolen something belonging to a patient yourself, but you observed someone else do so and failed to report the fact. Of what crime are you guilty?

_____

6. A visitor asks you if her father really has cancer. How should you respond?

_____

7. Unwelcome sexual advances and sexual behavior constitute _____.

8. Abuse is any act that is _____ and causes harm to the patient.

9. A door that is shut against a patient's will when the patient is confined to bed is a form of _____.

True/False

Mark the following true or false by circling T or F.

1. T F It is the responsibility of a nursing assistant to determine whether a patient has been abused.

2. T F A nursing assistant who reports bruises or wounds noted on a patient is acting properly.

3. T F Signs of poor personal hygiene and a change in personality may indicate abuse.

4. T F Most abuse originates in feelings of frustration and fatigue.

5. T F For help in reducing personal stress, request counseling through an employee assistance program.

6. T F Separation of a patient may be permitted if it is part of a therapeutic plan to reduce agitation.

7. T F A nursing assistant may independently decide to isolate a patient.

8. T F In some states, a person who does not report abuse is held as guilty as the actual abuser.

Complete the Chart

Place an X in the appropriate space to show which type of abuse has taken place.

Action	Verbal Abuse	Sexual Abuse	Psychological Abuse	Physical Abuse
1. Touching a patient in a sexual way	——	——	——	——
2. Using obscene gestures	——	——	——	——
3. Raising your voice in anger	——	——	——	——
4. Teasing a patient	——	——	——	——
5. Handling a patient roughly	——	——	——	——
6. Making threats	——	——	——	——
7. Making fun of the patient	——	——	——	——
8. Ridiculing a patient's behavior	——	——	——	——
9. Suggesting that the patient engage in sexual acts with you	——	——	——	——
10. Hitting a patient	——	——	——	——
11. Leaving the patient in bed when she asks repeatedly to get up	——	——	——	——
12. Holding an alert, cooperative patient down while the nurse performs a dressing change	——	——	——	——
13. Seating an alert patient at a table with three confused patients, rather than seating her in an empty spot at a table with three alert patients	——	——	——	——
14. Wiping inside a female patient's vagina with a washcloth while doing perineal care	——	——	——	——
15. Turning a patient roughly and abruptly	——	——	——	——
16. Saying, "If you don't stop using the call signal so much, I am not going to bring your lunch tray"	——	——	——	——
17. Unplugging the patient's call signal because she is making too many minor requests	——	——	——	——
18. Deliberately arousing a confused male patient when applying a condom catheter	——	——	——	——

DEVELOPING GREATER INSIGHT

Read the situations below and determine if the nursing assistant's behavior was negligent. Why or why not?

1. Mrs. Levitt has an order for side rails when in bed. The nursing assistant left the rails down and left the room. Mrs. Levitt tried to get up without help and fell, breaking her hip.

   _____

   _____

   _____

   _____

2. The nursing assistant discovers a large wet spot in the hallway while responding to a call light at the far end of the hall. The assistant walks around the puddle, goes to the patient's room, and answers the call light. When leaving the room, the assistant hears a commotion, and sees a visitor on the floor near the puddle, bleeding from the head. Several staff are attending him.

   _____

   _____

   _____

   _____

3. According to the care plan, Mrs. Wetzel may be up in her room as desired. When you left the room 40 minutes ago, she was sitting in a chair reading the newspaper. You hear a noise and check on the patient. You find her on the floor. She says, "I fell."

   _____

   _____

   _____

   _____

4. Jennifer Gonsalves is a 33-year-old patient who had a total abdominal hysterectomy. You are to check her surgical dressing every 2 hours. You are running late. Two hours and 25 minutes after the last check, you find a large spot of blood on the dressing.

   _____

   _____

   _____

5. Joseph Zeleski is a confused patient from the nursing home who wanders. You are to monitor his whereabouts to ensure that he does not leave the unit. You are also assigned to give another patient a bed bath. When you have finished, Mr. Zeleski is nowhere to be found. A search reveals that he left the unit, fell off the curb on the sidewalk, and is lying on the driveway moaning.

   _____

   _____

   _____

Scientific Principles

Medical Terminology and Body Organization

OBJECTIVES

After completing this unit, you will be able to:

- Spell and define terms.
- Write the abbreviations commonly used in health care facilities.
- Describe the organization of the body, from simple to complex.
- Name four types of tissues and their characteristics.
- Name and locate major organs as parts of body systems, using proper anatomic terms.
- State the location and functions of each body system.

UNIT SUMMARY

Medical terminology is developed by arranging and combining word parts. It is a language used by personnel in health care facilities. The words are formed of:

- Word roots
- Prefixes at the beginning of words
- Suffixes at the end of words
- Combining forms referring to body parts and medical actions

- Abbreviations (usually letters)

The human body is organized into:

- Various kinds of cells
- Four basic tissue types
- Many organs
- 10 systems

Each contributes in a special way to the total structure and physiology of the body. A careful study of the healthy body and its organization provides a foundation for learning about your own body and the bodies of your patients. Learning medical terminology will improve your understanding, help you communicate more effectively in the health care setting, and improve your accuracy in reporting and documenting your observations.

NURSING ASSISTANT ALERT

Action	Benefit
Analyze medical and scientific terms.	Improves comprehension. Increases vocabulary. Improves communication skills.
Practice using combining forms.	Increases verbal and written skills.
Study the anatomy and physiology of the body.	Improves understanding of normal body structure and functions.
Learn proper names for body parts.	Allows more accurate communication of observations.

ACTIVITIES

Vocabulary Exercise

Define the words in the spaces provided.

1. prefix

   WorD Part added at the beginning of a word

2. suffix

   Word Part added at the ending of a word

3. abbreviation

   Shorten Form of a word

4. combining forms

   Coming the word root and Vowel

5. word root

   ★ It's always the Part of the body
   ★ Condition that is being treated.

Completion

Complete the statements in the spaces provided.

1. Name the book, other than your text, that would be most helpful in studying medical terms.

   _____

2. Underline the <u>root</u> in each of the following words and give a definition of the word.

   Example: <u>abdomin</u>al pertaining to the abdomen

   a. adenoma *adeno Pertaining to gland*

   b. colectomy _____

   c. craniotomy *cranio Pertaining Skull*

d. dentist _____

e. hysterectomy _____

f. myalgia _____

g. nephrolithiasis _____

h. pneumonectomy _____

i. thoracotomy _____

j. urinometer _____

3. Underline the <u>prefix</u> in each of the following words and give a definition of the prefix.

   Example: <u>neo</u>plasm   new

   a. asepsis _____

   b. bradycardia _____

   c. dysuria _____

   d. hypertension _____

   e. hypotension _____

   f. pandemic _____

   g. polyuria _____

   h. gerontology _____

   i. premenstrual _____

   j. tachycardia _____

4. Underline the <u>suffix</u> in each of the following words and give a definition of the suffix.

   Example: acro<u>megaly</u>   great

   a. appendectomy _____

   b. hepatitis _____

   c. electrocardiogram _____

   d. anemia _____

   e. tracheotomy _____

   f. hematology _____

   g. hemiplegia _____

   h. apnea _____

   i. otoscope _____

   j. proctoscopy _____

5. Listed below are five words not in your text. Define each and then check your accuracy with a medical dictionary.

   a. adenitis

   _____

   b. cardiopathy

   _____

   c. leukopenia

   _____

d. arthroscope

_____

e. cytomegaly

_____

6. Substitute one word for the underlined words in each of the following statements.

Example: The patient experienced <u>pus in the urine</u>.   pyuria

a. There was <u>sugar in the urine</u>. _____

b. The patient made an appointment with a <u>physician who specializes in female diseases</u>.

_____

c. The nurse performed a <u>puncture in a vein</u> and drew blood.

_____

d. The patient has an <u>incision made into the trachea</u> to ease breathing.

_____

e. The patient had a <u>tumor composed mainly of fibrous tissue</u> removed from her uterus.

_____

f. The patient was receiving chemotherapy for cancer, which caused <u>depression of all her cell levels</u>.

_____

g. The nursing assistant listened with the stethoscope to the patient's heart. She found <u>the heart rate was slow</u>.

_____

h. The medication did not seem to help the patient's <u>high blood pressure</u>.

_____

i. The postoperative diagnosis was <u>removal of a lung</u>. _____

j. The patient complained of pain <u>under the stomach</u>. _____

7. Explain the following diagnoses.

a. thrombosis

_____

b. pyogenic infection

_____

c. pneumonitis

_____

d. cystitis

_____

e. mastitis

_____

8. Write the name of the body part indicated by the abbreviation.

a. abd _____

b. bld _____

c. G.I. _____

d. AX _____

e. GU _____

f. vag _____

g. sh _____

Matching

Match the letters on the left with the medical diagnosis on the right.

1. _____ AIDS   a. fracture

2. _____ CHF   b. transient ischemic attack

3. _____ CVA   c. hepatitis C virus

4. _____ Fx   d. multiple sclerosis

5. _____ TIA   e. acquired immune deficiency syndrome

6. _____ MI   f. sexually transmitted disease

7. _____ HCV   g. cerebrovascular accident

8. _____ KS   h. Kaposi's sarcoma

9. _____ STD   i. myocardial infarction

10. _____ MS   j. congestive heart failure

Abbreviations

The following is a list of abbreviations you will see relating to orders and patient care. Write your understanding of each abbreviation.

1. a. amb. ad lib. _____

   b. urine to lab ASAP _____

   c. BR only _____

   d. ck drsg freq _____

   e. OOB daily _____

   f. position HOB 45° _____

   g. discontinue cl liq diet _____

   h. SSE prn _____

   i. NPO preop _____

2. Write the names of the following hospital departments.

   a. CS _____

   b. EENT _____

   c. PT _____

   d. ICCU _____

   e. ED _____

   f. PAR _____

g. Peds _____

h. DR _____

i. OR _____

j. Lab _____

3. Write the appropriate abbreviation for the time indicated.

a. before meals _____

b. twice daily _____

c. morning _____

d. three times daily _____

e. after meals _____

f. immediately _____

g. four times a day _____

h. while awake _____

i. every hour _____

j. night _____

4. Write the word for each of the following measurements.

a. $\overline{ss}$ _____

b. mL _____

c. lb _____

d. kg _____

e. L _____

Roman Numerals

Write the Roman numerals for each of the following numbers.

1. one _____

2. twelve _____

3. six _____

4. nine _____

5. four _____

Word Puzzle

Unscramble the medical terms and write them in the center of the star. Then define each term in the spaces provided.

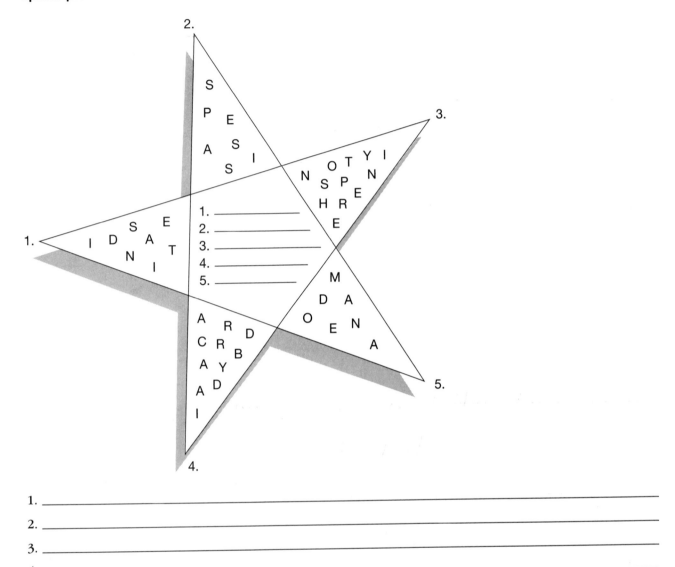

1. _____

2. _____

3. _____

4. _____

5. _____

Completion

Follow the directions for answering these questions.

1. Complete the organizational pattern of the body.

cells → _____ → _____ → systems

2. There are four tissue types. Write their names and list their functions.

a. _____

_____

b. _____

_____

c. _____

_____

d. _____

_____

3. Select the proper directional term from the list provided for each area indicated. Then color the organs as specified in the list.

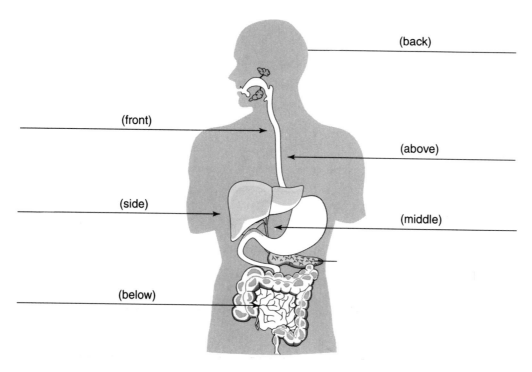

anterior	medial
inferior	posterior
lateral	superior

Organ Colors

Appendix—brown

Liver—green

Small intestine—red

Pancreas—yellow

Stomach—orange

4. Use the correct term to identify the relationships of the body parts listed by writing the correct answer in the space provided.

Answer

a. breasts   (anterior)   (posterior)   _____

b. heels   (anterior)   (posterior)   _____

c. toes   (anterior)   (posterior)   _____

d. buttocks   (anterior)   (posterior)   _____

e. abdomen   (anterior)   (posterior)   _____

f. breast related to legs   (superior)   (inferior)   _____

g. ankles related to legs   (superior)   (inferior)   _____

h. head related to toes   (superior)   (inferior)   _____

i. hips related to breasts   (superior)   (inferior)   _____

j. thumb related to little finger (medial)   (lateral)   _____

5. Another term for anterior is _____.

6. Another term for posterior is _____.

7. Write the proper abbreviations for abdominal regions.

   a. Patient A is complaining of pain in the area of his appendix. You properly identify this area as the

   _____.

   b. Patient B is complaining of discomfort in the area of his stomach. You properly identify this area as the

   _____.

   c. Patient C is complaining of pain over the region of his liver. You properly identify this area as the

   _____.

   d. Patient D is complaining of pain over the region where the lower descending colon is located. You properly

   identify this area as the _____.

Matching

Place the organs in the proper systems.

Organ

1. _____ Spleen

2. _____ Brain

3. _____ Breasts

4. _____ Kidneys

5. _____ Ureters

6. _____ Vagina

7. _____ Bones

8. _____ Heart

9. _____ Pituitary gland

10. _____ Joints

System

a. Cardiovascular

b. Endocrine

c. Digestive

d. Integumentary

e. Skeletal

f. Muscular

g. Nervous

h. Reproductive

i. Respiratory

j. Urinary

Match the function and the system.

Function

11. _____ Transports, absorbs food

12. _____ Regulates body processes through hormones

13. _____ Fulfills sexual needs

14. _____ Brings in oxygen

15. _____ Forms walls of some organs

16. _____ Eliminates liquid wastes

17. _____ Acts as levers in movement

18. _____ Produces hormones to regulate body functions

19. _____ Carries oxygen and nutrients to cells

20. _____ Coordinates body activities through nervous impulses

System

a. Cardiovascular

b. Endocrine

c. Digestive

d. Integumentary

e. Skeletal

f. Muscular

g. Nervous

h. Reproductive

i. Respiratory

j. Urinary

DEVELOPING GREATER INSIGHT

Label the following diagrams:

1.

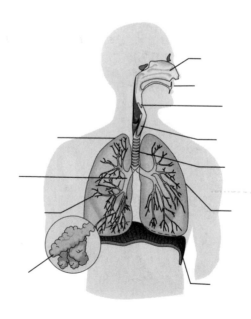

2.

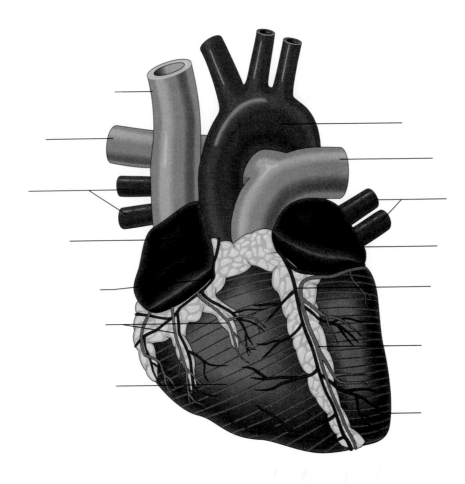

3.

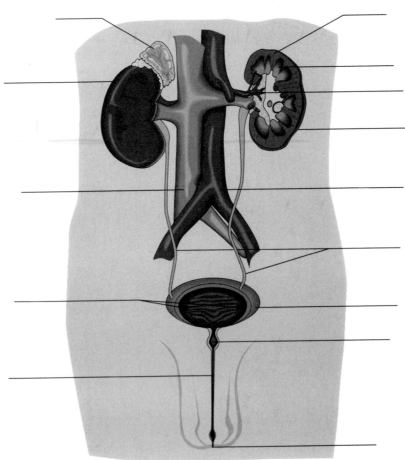

4.

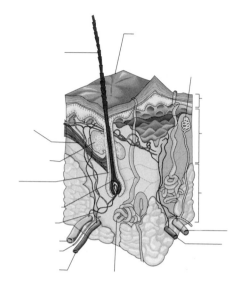

5.

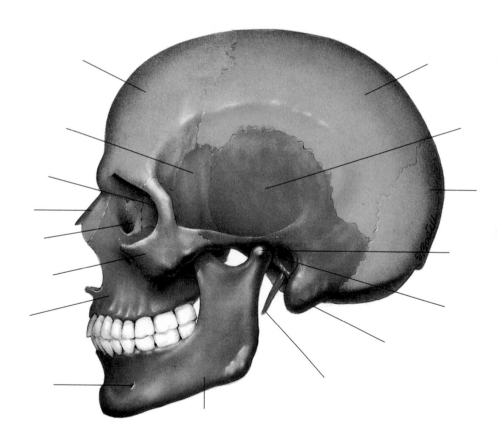

6.

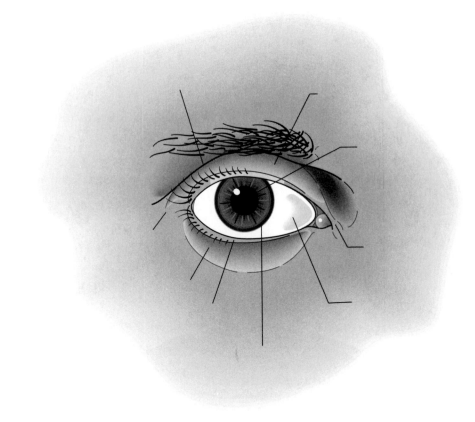

7.

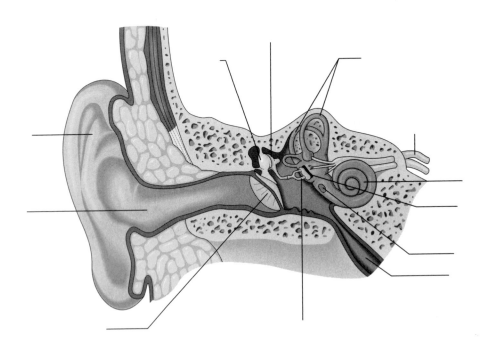

8.

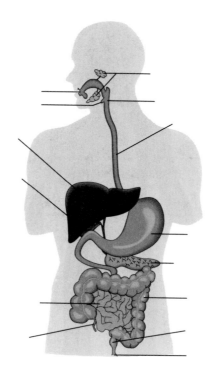

9.

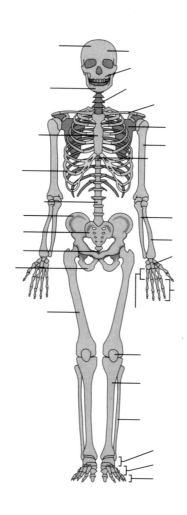

10.

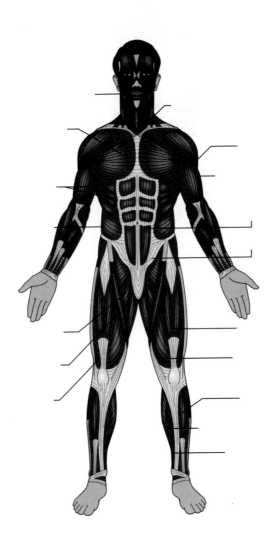

11.

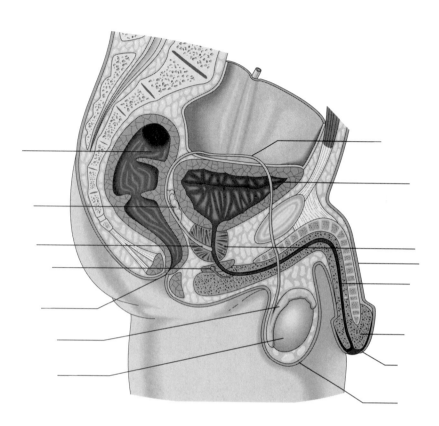

12.

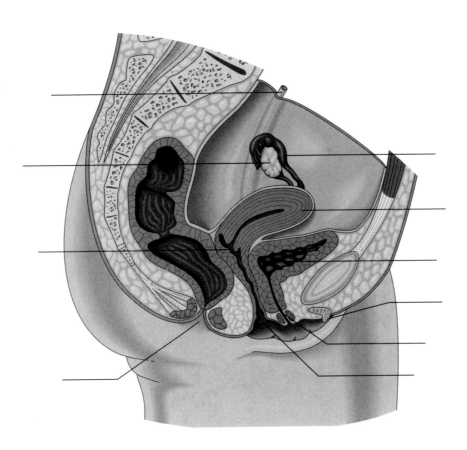

Classification of Disease

After completing this unit, you will be able to:

- Spell and define terms.
- Define disease and list some possible causes.
- Distinguish between signs and symptoms.
- List ways in which a diagnosis is made.
- Recognize alternative medicine and therapies.
- Understand the body's natural defenses against disease.

UNIT SUMMARY

Disease is any change from a healthy state. Disease takes many forms and has many causes. A variety of factors influence promotion of resistance to disease. Specific terms are used when discussing disease, such as:

- Etiology
- Signs and symptoms
- Prognosis
- Risk factors
- Predisposing factors

Diagnoses are made using laboratory and other diagnostic tests.

Types of therapy include:

- Surgery
- Chemotherapy
- Radiation
- Supportive care

Body defenses include:

- Unbroken skin
- Mucous membranes
- Mucus
- Acidity of secretions
- White blood cells
- Inflammation
- Immune response

NURSING ASSISTANT ALERT

Action	Benefit
Observe signs and symptoms carefully.	Accurate information is gathered.
Report observations promptly.	Prompt and proper action can be taken.

ACTIVITIES

Vocabulary Exercise

Complete the puzzle by filling in the missing letters of words found in this unit. Use the definitions to help you discover these words.

1. naming the disease process	1.	D — — — — — — —
2. tests that penetrate the body	2.	— — — — I — —
3. seen by others	3.	S — — — —
4. option to regular health care	4.	— — — E — — — — —
5. product given to prevent development of disease	5.	— A — — — —
6. outcome of a disease	6.	— — — — — S — —
7. treatment	7.	— — E — — —

Definitions

1. Define *disease*.

   _____

2. Define *etiology*.

   _____

Matching

For each observation, mark whether it is a sign (a) or a symptom (b).

Observation   **Classification**

1. _____ rash   a. sign

2. _____ nausea   b. symptom

3. _____ pain

4. _____ elevated temperature

5. _____ increased pulse rate

6. _____ vomiting

7. _____ flushed skin

8. _____ dizziness

9. _____ itching

10. _____ anxious feelings

Completion

Complete the statements in the spaces provided.

1. The body has special natural defenses. List five.

   a. _____

   b. _____

   c. _____

   d. _____

   e. _____

2. List four basic forms of therapy.

   a. _____

   b. _____

   c. _____

   d. _____

3. List five signs and symptoms of acute inflammation.

   a. _____

   b. _____

   c. _____

   d. _____

   e. _____

Clinical Situations

Briefly describe how a nursing assistant should react to each of the following situations.

1. Your neighbor Elizabeth Simmons tells you she has a lump in her breast but she has told no one else.

_____

_____

_____

2. Mrs. Torres has a cerebral thrombus. Follow the maze to identify its location.

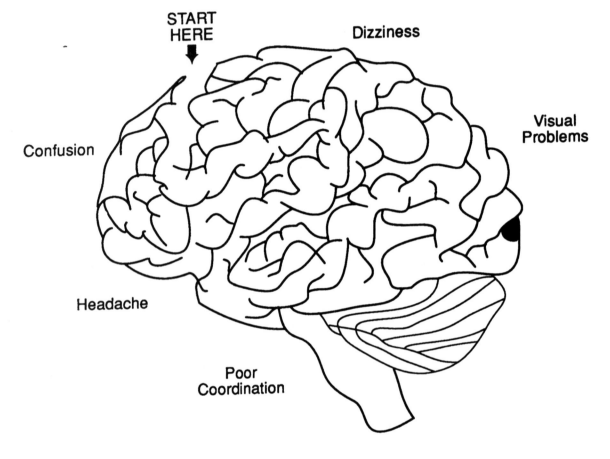

   a. What part of the body is affected? _____

   b. Define these words:

     cerebral _____

     thrombus _____

DEVELOPING GREATER INSIGHT

Complete the puzzle using the clues below. Write the missing words on the line with the clues below.

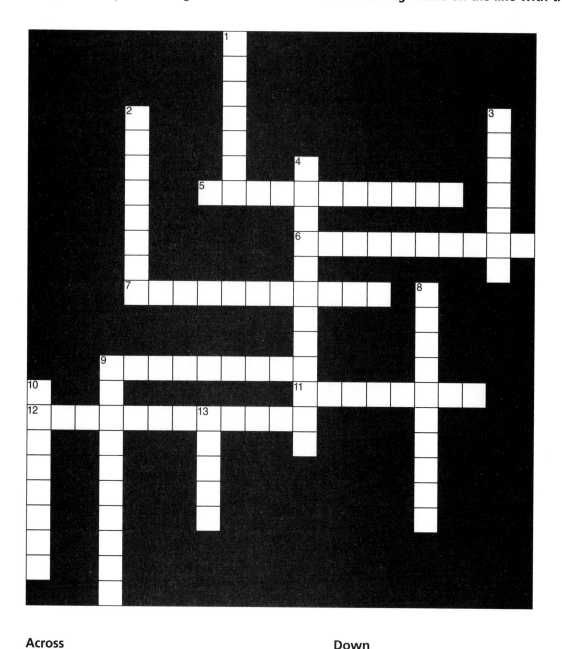

Across

5 _____ health care practices and products are options to regular health care.

6 _____ studies give the physician valuable information for naming the disease and planning the treatment.

7 _____ studies are done without breaking the skin or damaging body tissue.

9 Mucous _____ secrete a sticky substance that traps foreign particles, preventing them from invading the body.

Down

1 Making a _____ diagnosis is the process of identifying and naming a disease.

2 _____ skin protects the outside of the body from invading pathogens.

3 A person with _____ disease may have periods when signs and symptoms are marked and periods when the disease is less pronounced.

4 _____ factors to disease are conditions that may contribute to the development of illness.

11 _____ tests penetrate body surfaces.

12 An acute _____ of a chronic disease is when the severity of signs and symptoms increases.

8 _____ care is a type of therapy that supports the patient's body in its attempt to return to health.

9 Normal body defenses act as _____ barriers to protect a person against disease.

10 Body _____ provide a natural line of protection from disease.

13 An _____ disease develops suddenly, progresses rapidly, and lasts for a predictable period.

Basic Human Needs and Communication

UNIT **7**

Communication Skills

OBJECTIVES

After completing this unit, you will be able to:

- Spell and define terms.
- List the four components of an effective message.
- Explain the types of verbal and nonverbal communication.
- Identify four tools of communication for staff members.
- State the guidelines for communicating effectively with patients.

UNIT SUMMARY

Communication is a two-way process of sharing information. Communications must be clear between yourself and patients, coworkers, and those in authority. Communications are sent through:

- Oral or verbal language
- Body language
- Written messages

Special communication techniques must be used when communicating with patients who have impaired hearing or vision, patients who are disoriented, and patients who have certain medical problems, such as aphasia (loss of normal ability to speak or understand).

NURSING ASSISTANT ALERT

Action	Benefit
Communicate effectively with coworkers.	Ensures that accurate information is transmitted properly. Ensures that the safest care will be given.
Communicate effectively with patients.	Ensures that patients' needs will be recognized and understood. Means that directions will be properly understood by patients.
Communicate effectively with families and visitors.	Conveys a feeling of welcome and security to family members and visitors.

ACTIVITIES

Vocabulary Exercise

Define the following by selecting the correct term from the list provided.

body language	communication
culture	feedback
nonverbal communication	paraphrasing
receiver	sender
symbols	verbal communication

1. Objects used to represent something else   _____

2. Restating and confirming your understanding of a message   _____

3. Spoken words   _____

4. The person for whom the message is intended   _____

5. The person who is speaking or communicating the message   _____

6. Communicating through body movements   _____

7. Customs, languages, and traditions of specific groups of people _____

8. Communicating without oral speech   _____

9. Confirmation that a message was received as intended   _____

10. Exchanging information   _____

Completion

Complete the statements in the spaces provided.

1. Describe the purpose of each of the following.

   a. Employee's personnel handbook

   _____

   b. Disaster manual

   _____

   c. Procedure manual

   _____

d. Nursing policy manual

_____

e. Assignment

_____

2. List types of information that might be learned in a staff development class.

a. _____

b. _____

c. _____

d. _____

3. Four things are needed for successful communication. They are:

a. _____

b. _____

c. _____

d. _____

4. List six ways in which people communicate without using words.

a. _____

b. _____

c. _____

d. _____

e. _____

f. _____

5. State five ways you can improve communications with patients.

a. _____

b. _____

c. _____

d. _____

e. _____

6. List ways a message can be sent through body language.

a. _____

b. _____

c. _____

d. _____

e. _____

f. _____

Complete the following statements by selecting the correct term(s) from the list provided.

anger	articulate	caring	clearly	cover
cues	double	hand	happiness	hearing
identify	lengthy	lightly	loudness (volume)	objects
one	patronizing	sadness	see	slang
specific	substitutes	talking	tone	

1. When communicating verbally, remember to

   a. Control the _____ of your voice.

   b. Control your voice _____.

   c. Be aware of the way you _____.

   d. Avoid _____ meanings or cultural meanings.

   e. Not use informal language or _____.

2. Loudness and tone of your voice can convey a message of

   a. _____

   b. _____

   c. _____

   d. _____

3. Complete the nursing organizational chart using the following names and titles.

   rehabilitation aides   nurse manager   staff nurses

   nursing assistants   unit secretaries   patient care technicians

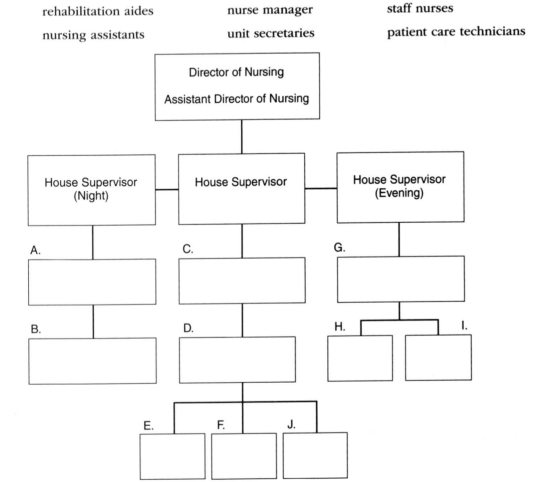

4. Your verbal message is interpreted like this:

_____% words

+ _____% tone of voice

+ _____% facial expression, body language, gestures

_____

= 100% total communication

Complete the form provided

5. Father Duchene, the priest at St. Gregory's Catholic Church, called at 10:00 AM on November 11 to ask how Mrs. Riley was feeling. He wanted to speak to the nurse manager, Mr. Burke, who was busy at the time and unavailable. Father Duchene asked that the nurse manager return his call. His telephone number is 683-4972. How do you communicate this information? Complete the following form to demonstrate your understanding of the proper way to do this task.

To	☐ URGENT
Date _____ Time _____	A.M. P.M.

WHILE YOU WERE OUT

From _____

Of _____

Phone _____

Area Code / Number / Ext.

Telephoned		Please call	
Came to see you		Wants to see you	
Returned your call		Will call again	

Message _____
_____
_____
_____
_____
_____
_____

Signed _____

Yes or No

Do the words and the body language send the same message? Circle Y for yes or N for no.

1. Y N Wendy rubs her head with her hand and tells you she does not have a headache.

2. Y N Ellen sits with her arms and legs crossed, has turned her wheelchair toward the window, and tells you she is happy to meet her new daughter-in-law.

3. Y N Aimee makes a face when you feed her and says she hates chocolate pudding.

4. Y N Mary appears on duty with dirty shoes and untidy hair and says she is proud to be a nursing assistant.

5. Y N Chris keeps moving about the room and rubbing her hands together and says she feels calm about her transfer to another facility.

6. Y N Nichole says she is interested in her patients. She often looks out the window and seldom makes eye contact when patients speak.

7. Y N Carrie and Terry claim to care about patients and often talk "over" them as they work together giving care.

8. Y N Tim describes himself as a caring nursing assistant. He often interrupts patients when they are talking.

9. Y N Fernando says he is sensitive to patients' feelings and stands about six feet away when conversing with them.

10. Y N Grace is careful to show caring by never discussing personal activities with other staff members in the presence of patients.

CLINICAL SITUATIONS

Read the following situations and answer the questions.

1. Mr. Fedin is an immigrant from Poland. Prior to his stroke, he spoke English. Now he speaks only in Polish. His family says he is confused, and that he is not making sense when he speaks in his native tongue. At times he seems to understand when you speak to him in English, but he responds in Polish. Communication with him has been particularly difficult for the staff. You are assigned to care for him.

   a. List several approaches to use when communicating with this patient in English.

   _____

   _____

   b. How will you learn about special methods and techniques used to communicate with this patient?

   _____

   _____

   c. Will raising your voice help Mr. Fedin understand?

   _____

   _____

   d. What are two nonverbal communication techniques that may be useful with this patient?

   _____

   _____

Observation, Reporting, and Documentation

OBJECTIVES

After completing this unit, you will be able to:

- Spell and define terms.
- List the components of the nursing process.
- Describe the purpose of the care plan.
- Explain the nursing assistant's responsibilities for each component of the nursing process.
- Describe two observations to make for each body system.
- List three times when oral reports are given.
- Describe the information given when reporting.
- State the purpose of the patient's medical record.
- Explain the rules for documentation.
- State the purpose of the HIPAA laws.

UNIT SUMMARY

Patient-focused care is carried out most effectively when communications are accurately passed between coworkers and between caregivers and patients. This is achieved by:

- Following the nursing process
- Developing an individual care plan for each patient
- Proper documentation and reporting

The nursing process has five steps, and nursing assistants make a valuable contribution to each. The four steps are:

1. Assessment
2. Problem identification
3. Planning
4. Implementation
5. Evaluation

NURSING ASSISTANT ALERT

Action	Benefit
Observe and report carefully.	Alerts nurse to changes in patient's condition so proper care can be given.
Document accurately.	Keeps staff informed of patient's status.
Follow nursing care plan faithfully.	Ensures proper care for the individual patient.

ACTIVITIES

Vocabulary Exercise

Each line has four different spellings of a word from this unit. Circle the correctly spelled word.

1. assesment	ascesment	accessment	assessment
2. charing	charting	sharting	chartting
3. process	procese	prosess	processe
4. graphic	grephic	grafic	graffic
5. obsavation	obserbation	observation	observachian
6. communication	comunication	cummunication	communikation
7. cardex	Kardex	cadex	kardix
8. evaleation	evaloation	evaluation	eveluation

Completion

Complete the following statements in the spaces provided.

1. The five steps of the nursing process and their definitions are:

Step	Definition
a. _____	_____
b. _____	_____
c. _____	_____
d. _____	_____
e. _____	_____

2. What are three types of information you will find on the care plan?

   a. _____

   b. _____

   c. _____

3. The nursing diagnosis is a statement of _____

   _____

4. The nursing diagnosis reflects

   a. _____

   b. _____

   c. _____

   d. _____

5. The nursing diagnosis provides the foundation for _____.

6. The nurse coordinates assessment with _____

   _____

7. The care plan is kept in a vertical storage file called a _____ or in the _____.

8. The intervention (approach) states

   a. _____

   b. _____

   c. _____

9. Nursing assistants are responsible for knowing when and _____

   the approach is to be carried out and for implementing the approach _____.

10. The final step in the nursing process is the _____.

11. The nursing assistant is responsible for reporting to the nurse when _____.

12. Critical pathways detail the:

    a. _____

    b. _____

13. The critical pathway lists nursing actions to _____.

Differentiation

Differentiate between signs and symptoms by writing each observation under the proper label in the spaces provided.

Sign	Symptom	Observation
1. _____	_____	nausea
2. _____	_____	vomiting
3. _____	_____	pain
4. _____	_____	restlessness
5. _____	_____	dizziness
6. _____	_____	cold, clammy skin
7. _____	_____	incontinence
8. _____	_____	elevated blood pressure
9. _____	_____	anxiety
10. _____	_____	cough

Matching

Name the sense used to determine the following information.

1. _____ Body odor
2. _____ Radial pulse
3. _____ Wheezing when the patient breathes
4. _____ Comments from the patient
5. _____ Blood in urine
6. _____ A change in the way a patient walks
7. _____ Warmth of the patient's skin
8. _____ Bruises
9. _____ Lump under the patient's skin
10. _____ The patient crying

a. eyes

b. ears

c. smell

d. touch

Matching

Match the observation on the left with the system on the right to which it most relates.

Observation

1. _____ curled up in bed
2. _____ disoriented as to time and place
3. _____ regular pulse
4. _____ elevated blood pressure
5. _____ jaundiced (yellow) skin
6. _____ skin warm to touch
7. _____ difficulty breathing
8. _____ unable to respond with words
9. _____ cloudy urine
10. _____ site of injection hot and red
11. _____ difficulty passing stool
12. _____ belching frequently following a meal
13. _____ vaginal discharge
14. _____ drowsy, not responding well
15. _____ nauseated, vomited small amount of clear fluid

System

a. circulatory

b. integumentary

c. muscular

d. skeletal

e. nervous

f. respiratory

g. digestive

h. endocrine

i. reproductive

j. urinary

Multiple Choice

Select the one best answer for each question.

1. To find information about care to be given to an individual patient, you should consult the

   a. patient's medical chart.
   b. procedure manual.
   c. patient care plan.
   d. nursing policy manual.

2. For the most up-to-date information about the patient's condition, check the

   a. patient's medical chart.
   b. nursing policy manual.
   c. procedure manual.
   d. patient care plan.

3. The patient's chart

   a. is not a permanent document.
   b. is a legal document.
   c. is properly written in pencil.
   d. may be used only while the patient is in the hospital facility.

4. When you report off duty, your report should include

   a. details on how your day went.
   b. the care you gave each patient.
   c. comments about patients not in your care.
   d. observations on how well the staff got along.

5. Nursing assistants may document on the

   a. physician's order sheet.
   b. consultant record.
   c. dietary record.
   d. flow sheet.

6. Charting must

   a. be about all the patients in one room.
   b. address problems listed in the patient care plan.
   c. include the wishes of the family.
   d. be documented in subjective terms.

7. When charting,

   a. use objective statements.
   b. use complete sentences.
   c. make up abbreviations to save space.
   d. round off times to the closest hour.

8. Your patient has a kidney condition. You should note

   a. rate of respirations.
   b. edema.
   c. vaginal drainage.
   d. appetite.

9. Your patient has a digestive problem. You should note

   a. color of sputum.
   b. orientation to time.
   c. belching.
   d. lumps.

10. Your patient has a heart problem. You should note

    a. regularity of pulse.
    b. mental status.
    c. nasal drainage.
    d. ability to walk.

Matching

Match the regular time and its equivalent in international time.

Regular Time	**International Time**
1. _____ 12:30 AM	a. 1230
2. _____ 7:15 AM	b. 1915
3. _____ 2:30 PM	c. 0800
4. _____ 8 PM	d. 1430
5. _____ 4:30 PM	e. 2000
	f. 0030
	g. 0715
	h. 1630

Completion

Complete each statement as it relates to charting by selecting the proper word from those provided.

blank	clearly	color	completely	entry
error	patient	sequence	spell	title

1. Fill out new headings _____.

2. Use the correct _____ of ink.

3. Date and time each _____.

4. Chart entries in correct _____.

5. Print or write _____.

6. _____ each word correctly.

7. Leave no _____ spaces between entries.

8. Do not use the word _____.

9. Sign each entry with your first initial, last name, and _____.

10. Make a correction by drawing one line through the entry and printing the word _____ on the line with your initials.

Short Answer

Fill in brief answers in the spaces provided.

1. Fill in the blanks in the diagram. Explain the difference between nursing diagnosis and medical diagnosis.

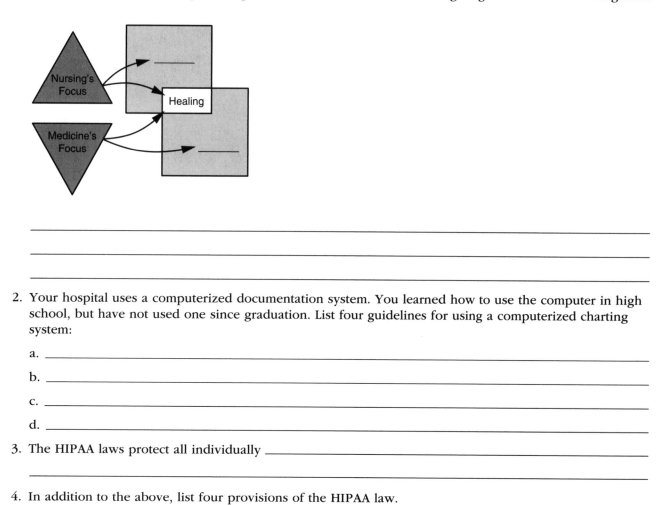

_____

_____

_____

2. Your hospital uses a computerized documentation system. You learned how to use the computer in high school, but have not used one since graduation. List four guidelines for using a computerized charting system:

   a. _____

   b. _____

   c. _____

   d. _____

3. The HIPAA laws protect all individually _____

   _____

4. In addition to the above, list four provisions of the HIPAA law.

   a. _____

   b. _____

   c. _____

   d. _____

Clinical Situations

Answer the following questions in regard to this patient's care.

Robert Gonzales is 62 years of age. He has had a stroke. He shows right-side weakness, alteration in cerebral tissue perfusion, and aphasia. The nurse has instructed you to assist with all ADLs. The patient showers. Vital signs are to be checked T.I.D.

1. How many times each day will you measure the patient's vital signs?

   _____

2. What kind of help might this patient need with ADLs?

   _____

3. What particular safety measure must you take during the shower?

_____

4. What problem does the aphasia cause?

_____

5. Explain the meanings of the following conditions.

a. right-side weakness _____

_____

b. alteration in cerebral tissue perfusion _____

_____

6. Will raising your voice help Mr. Gonzales understand? Why or why not?

_____

_____

7. List two observations of the nervous system that you will monitor in this patient.

a. _____

b. _____

DEVELOPING GREATER INSIGHT

Your unit has an open nurses' station. You notice a patient's family member standing around the corner near the station during report. Several times you have observed him near the chart rack when the station was unattended.

1. Is this a potential problem?

2. Why or why not?

3. What action will you take, if any?

4. You must print your notes at the end of the shift and place them on the chart. You accidentally printed 25 pages of unnecessary notes on Mr. Emery's chart. What will you do?

Meeting Basic Human Needs

After completing this unit, you will be able to:

- Spell and define terms.
- Describe the stages of human growth and development.
- List five physical needs of patients.
- Define self-esteem.
- List nursing assistant actions to ensure that patients have the opportunity for intimacy.
- Explain why cultural and spiritual beliefs influence patients' psychological responses.
- List some guidelines to assist patients in meeting their spiritual needs.

UNIT SUMMARY

Individuals develop at varying rates. There are, however, some well-defined developmental stages through which each person passes.

- Certain developmental skills are characteristically acquired at certain stages of life—from birth to death. A person's success in mastering these skills affects the progress of his development.

- Regardless of developmental level, people have common basic emotional and physical needs.

- The nursing staff must be sensitive to the influence of culture on the expression of individual needs.

- The way in which these needs are expressed varies, especially when a person is ill.

- The nursing staff must be sensitive to patients' individual needs. They must find ways of successfully providing for them.

NURSING ASSISTANT ALERT

Action	Benefit
Recognize that age groups differ in levels of development.	Each patient will be treated as an individual.
Accept patients as unique individuals with basic needs.	Care plans will be developed that consider and meet personal needs.

ACTIVITIES

Vocabulary Exercise

Unscramble the words introduced in this unit and define them. Select terms from the list provided.

continuum   growth   preadolescence   development

intimacy   sexuality   reflex   neonate

1. T E N O A N E _____

2. C E C A E N R E L D O P E S _____

3. N U C T O I N M U _____

4. W G O R H T _____

5. P O N L E E V D T E M _____

6. T I M A C I N Y _____

7. X E F E L R _____

8. U X A L I T S E Y _____

Fill in the Blank

Indicate which child is demonstrating appropriate behavior for his or her age group by marking A for appropriate or I for inappropriate.

1. _____ Scott, 16, is receiving an IV and is talking to Patty, 17, who is 2 days postoperative following an appendectomy.

2. _____ Bobbi, age 13, is stringing beads to make a bracelet.

3. _____ Felicia, age 8, and Kimmie, 11, are playing Pokémon Monopoly.

4. _____ Tommy, 14, and Brian, 15, are playing with wooden cars and trucks.

5. _____ Jonnie, 2½, is playing with blocks near the older boys.

6. _____ Dona, age 3, is sitting near Jonnie, pushing different-shaped blocks through the precut holes in a plastic ball.

Matching

Match the proper term on the right with the explanation of sexual expression on the left.

1. _____ sexual attraction to members of both sexes

2. _____ self-stimulation for sexual pleasure

3. _____ sexual attraction between members of the same sex

4. _____ sexual attraction to members of the opposite sex

a. masturbation

b. homosexuality

c. bisexuality

d. heterosexuality

Completion

Complete the statements in the spaces provided.

1. The stages of growth and development refer to the _____ that must be mastered before moving on to the next stage.

2. Jimmy Hinkle is 12 months old. He weighs 16 pounds and is 26 inches tall. He weighed 8 pounds at birth. You know that this is _____ than average for his chronological age.

3. The average vocabulary of a 2-year-old is about _____words.

4. Five characteristics of early adulthood include:

   a. _____

   b. _____

   c. _____

   d. _____

   e. _____

5. The sandwich generation of middle age refers to _____

   _____

6. Later maturity is characterized by a period of _____

   _____

Short Answer

1. Briefly explain Maslow's theory regarding human needs.

_____

_____

_____

_____

Clinical Situations

Briefly explain why you think the patient is acting this way and how you think the nursing assistant should react to the following situations.

1. Jeannie Hunt, age 16, has been diagnosed as having osteosarcoma of her right tibia. The prognosis is guarded and she has been scheduled for surgery to remove the right leg at mid-calf, to be followed by radiation. She asks to see the youth leader of her church.

   _____

   _____

2. Craig Martin, age 52, is recovering from a partial prostatectomy. He is complaining loudly about his care, the food, and the other patients in the room.

_____

_____

3. Lucy Wong, age 26, is having difficulty sleeping at bedtime. She is in your care.

_____

_____

4. You are serving nourishments and find the door to Rudolph Baker's room closed.

_____

_____

5. You are assigned to care for the two male patients in Room 762. You have reason to believe that they may be lovers and another nursing assistant asks you what you know about their relationship.

_____

_____

6. Every time you enter Belinda Mitchell's room, she makes sexual advances to you and tries to find reasons to touch you.

_____

_____

RELATING TO THE NURSING PROCESS

Write the step of the nursing process that is related to the nursing assistant action.

Nursing Assistant Action	Nursing Process Step
1. The nursing assistant assists the mature adult to ambulate.	_____
2. The nursing assistant reports that the 18-month-old baby has difficulty sitting up.	_____
3. The nursing assistant reports that the teenager is still having periods of depression.	_____
4. The nursing assistant pads the oxygen cannula to reduce irritation behind the patient's ears.	_____
5. The nursing assistant informs the nurse of an approach that is effective for Mr. Kardashian's care plan. The nurse is happy to learn this information and adds it to the plan.	_____
6. Mrs. Spitzer is not responding to her nursing plan of care. She has a new area of skin breakdown. The nurse has assigned each team member to collect data and has scheduled a care conference.	_____

Comfort, Pain, Rest, and Sleep

OBJECTIVES

After completing this unit, you will be able to:

- Spell and define terms.
- Explain how loud noise affects patients and hospital staff.
- Explain why nursing comfort measures are important to patients' well-being.
- List six observations to make and report for patients having pain.
- State the purpose of the pain rating scale and briefly describe how a pain scale is used.
- Describe nursing assistant measures to increase comfort, relieve pain, and promote rest and sleep.

UNIT SUMMARY

- Everyone needs comfort, rest, and sleep for physical and emotional well-being, health, and wellness.

- Comfort is a state of physical and emotional well-being. When a patient is comfortable, she is calm and relaxed, and is not in pain or upset.

- Excessive noise causes many surprising problems, such as delayed healing, impaired immune function, and increased heart rate and blood pressure. Noise causes feelings of anxiety, but patients do not always associate noise with the distress they feel.

- Patients who do not sleep well at night may be dissatisfied with the facility and nursing care. Some become confused and agitated when they are deprived of sleep. Confused patients may wander to escape the noise.

- Noise also has a detrimental effect on staff performance. The Environmental Protection Agency (EPA) recommends that hospital noise levels not exceed 45 decibels during the day. The World Health Organization (WHO) recommended keeping noise levels below 35 decibels in facilities. A whisper is approximately 30 decibels. Normal conversation causes about 60 decibels of noise.

- The noisiest time of day is usually during shift change.

- Pain is a state of discomfort that is unpleasant. Pain signifies that something is wrong.

- Pain interferes with the patient's level of function and ability to do self-care. It negatively affects quality of life.

- Pain causes stress and anxiety, interfering with comfort, rest, and sleep.

- The patient's self-report of pain is the most accurate indicator of the existence and intensity of pain, and should be respected and believed.

- Patients' complaints of pain always require further intervention.

- Pain rating scales are communication tools that help with assessment and prevent caregivers from forming their own opinions about the level of the patient's pain. Pain scales prevent subjective opinions, provide consistency, eliminate some barriers to pain management, and give the patient a means of describing the pain accurately.

- Rest is a state of mental and physical comfort, calmness, and relaxation. Basic needs of hunger, thirst, elimination, and pain must be met before rest is possible.

- A patient who is resting may sit or lie down, or do things that are pleasant and relaxing.

- Sleep is a basic need that is met during a period of continuous or intermittent unconsciousness in which physical movements are decreased.

- Adequate sleep is necessary for the body and mind to function properly, and for healing to occur.

- Many factors, both within control and beyond control, affect patients' comfort, rest, and sleep.

- Care should be scheduled to allow uninterrupted sleep whenever possible.

- A major nursing assistant responsibility is to provide basic personal care and comfort measures to help relieve pain and promote comfort, rest, and sleep.

NURSING ASSISTANT ALERT

Action	Benefit
Ensure privacy, reduce noise, eliminate unpleasant odors, and adjust the temperature, lighting, and ventilation.	Reduces factors that cause discomfort over which the patient has no control.
Handle the patient gently, assist the patient to assume a comfortable position, use pillows and props for repositioning, give a backrub, and provide emotional support.	Helps the patient to relax and rest better. Enhances comfort.
Meet the patient's basic needs of hunger, thirst, elimination, pain relief, and good hygiene.	Removes or relieves factors that interfere with proper rest.
Schedule care to prevent awakening the patient during sleep.	Helps the patient to sleep well, facilitating rest and healing of both mind and body.

ACTIVITIES

Vocabulary Exercise

Complete the word search puzzle using the clues below. Write the name of the missing word on the line of each clue.

g	a	s	s	e	s	s	m	e	n	t	B
e	o	A	l	e	b	i	c	e	d	e	t
c	n	l	H	f	m	Q	J	Y	s	r	x
i	c	v	d	S	t	M	A	i	o	h	g
s	c	P	i	e	O	w	o	p	y	l	n
e	Y	F	c	r	n	n	e	O	H	X	i
g	n	l	y	e	o	r	C	M	Q	t	d
l	i	c	k	p	-	n	s	l	f	s	r
a	a	U	e	f	w	h	m	c	A	e	a
n	p	e	l	F	Q	o	H	e	a	r	u
a	l	e	p	T	W	n	U	M	n	l	g
s	s	c	o	m	f	o	r	t	l	e	

1. The _____ should be calm and quiet to promote rest.

2. The patient's _____-_____ is the most accurate and reliable indicator of the existence and intensity of pain.

3. The pain _____ scale is a tool for communication.

4. Pain medication _____

5. An unconscious, protective action, position, or movement to shield a painful or injured area _____

6. A state of physical and emotional well-being _____

7. A measure of noise _____

8. The _____ rule for pain relief is that whatever is painful to adults is painful to children unless proven otherwise.

9. According to Florence Nightingale, "Unnecessary _____ is the most cruel abuse of care which can be inflicted on either the sick or the well."

10. A pain _____ is used to measure the level and intensity of a patient's pain.

11. A period of continuous or intermittent unconsciousness in which physical movements are decreased _____

12. The Occupational Safety and Health Administration _____

13. A state of discomfort that is unpleasant for the patient _____

14. A state of mental and physical comfort, calmness, and relaxation _____

Short Answer

Briefly complete the following.

1. List eight factors that may interfere with a patient's ability to sleep.

   a. _____

   b. _____

   c. _____

   d. _____

   e. _____

   f. _____

   g. _____

   h. _____

2. List eight observations that you see, hear, feel, or smell that should be reported to the nurse regarding a patient's pain.

   a. _____

   b. _____

   c. _____

   d. _____

   e. _____

   f. _____

   g. _____

   h. _____

3. How is a patient's outward expression of pain affected by culture?

   _____

4. List at least eight factors that affect patients' comfort, rest, and sleep.

   a. _____

   b. _____

   c. _____

   d. _____

   e. _____

   f. _____

   g. _____

   h. _____

5. What is the purpose of the pain rating scale?

   _____

6. Why is using the pain rating scale a key to accurate pain evaluation?

   _____

7. Your patient uses the FACES pain scale. The nurse gave her pain medication an hour ago. The patient tells you that her pain is now number 4. You should:

_____

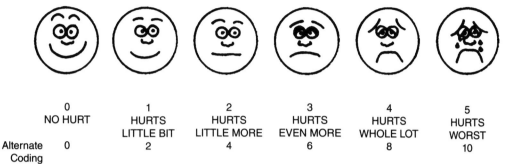

0 NO HURT	1 HURTS LITTLE BIT	2 HURTS LITTLE MORE	3 HURTS EVEN MORE	4 HURTS WHOLE LOT	5 HURTS WORST

Alternate   0   2   4   6   8   10
Coding

True/False

Mark the following true or false by circling T or F.

1. T   F   The nurse's assessment is always more accurate than a patient's self-report of pain intensity.

2. T   F   A patient must be lying in bed to rest properly.

3. T   F   Comfort is a state of well-being.

4. T   F   Elderly adults require less sleep than younger adults.

5. T   F   Elderly persons are often uncomfortable in a cool environment.

6. T   F   Phantom pain is psychological pain.

7. T   F   The body repairs itself during sleep.

8. T   F   A patient who is resting may pray or say the rosary.

9. T   F   If a patient is sick, hunger and thirst do not interfere with the ability to rest.

10. T   F   Lack of privacy may affect the patient's comfort and ability to rest.

11. T   F   According to the EPA, hospital noise should not exceed 138 decibels during the day.

12. T   F   Some patients believe that excessive noise is an invasion of their privacy.

13. T   F   Excessive noise has no effect on the stress level of staff.

14. T   F   Hospital workers must be active listeners for good communication.

15. T   F   Body language is not affected by pain.

16. T   F   A confused patient with garbled speech may be able to describe her pain accurately.

17. T   F   Because nurses assess pain, the nursing assistant need not bother learning about the pain scales the facility uses.

18. T   F   Unrelieved pain affects the patient's health.

19. T   F   Unrelieved pain may cause feelings of anxiety.

RELATING TO THE NURSING PROCESS

List 10 things the nursing assistant can do to enhance comfort, rest, and sleep and relieve pain.

1. _____
2. _____
3. _____
4. _____
5. _____
6. _____
7. _____
8. _____
9. _____
10. _____

DEVELOPING GREATER INSIGHT

Your patient, Mrs. Hernandez, has spinal stenosis and frequently complains of pain. The nurse alternates an injection for pain with an oral medication every 2 hours.

1. Mrs. Hernandez is laughing and visiting with her family. When you enter the room with fresh ice water, she tells you she is in pain. Can a patient who is laughing and visiting be having pain? Explain your answer.

_____
_____
_____

2. Mrs. Hernandez refuses her supper tray. She tells you she is in too much pain to eat. What action should you take?

_____
_____
_____

3. Mrs. Hernandez tells you that she feels better now, and would like to eat. The kitchen has closed for the evening. What action should you take?

_____
_____
_____

4. Why do you think that hunger, thirst, pain, and need to use the bathroom affect patients' comfort and ability to rest or sleep?

_____

_____

_____

_____

5. Mrs. Hernandez cannot sleep. She tells you that her low back really hurts. What nursing assistant measures can you take to make her more comfortable?

_____

_____

_____

_____

Developing Cultural Sensitivity

OBJECTIVES

After completing this unit, you will be able to:

- Spell and define terms.

- Name six major cultural groups in the United States.

- Describe ways major cultures may differ in family organization, communication, need for personal space, health practices, religion, and traditions.

- List ways the nursing assistant can help patients in practicing rituals appropriate to their cultures.

- State ways the nursing assistant can demonstrate appreciation of and sensitivity to persons from other cultures.

UNIT SUMMARY

Patients have a variety of cultural heritages. These heritages influence how individuals:

- Communicate

- React to health concerns

- View one another and the need for personal space

- Celebrate holidays

- Select foods

- Practice religions beliefs

Culture also may affect:

- The patient's beliefs about health, wellness, and illness

- The patient's hygienic practices

- How the patient reacts to illness

- The patient's expectations about how care should be given and by whom

- The patient's participation in self-care during times of illness

Six ethnic groups predominate in the United States. They are:

- Caucasian
- African American
- Hispanic
- Asian/Pacific
- Native American
- Middle Eastern/Arab

Nursing assistants must treat all patients as individuals and be sensitive to:

- The patient's acceptance of caregivers
- The amount of disrobing permitted
- The degree of touch that is comfortable

NURSING ASSISTANT ALERT

Action	Benefit
Learn as much as possible about a patient's culture.	Helps patients receive more personalized care.
Treat patients as individuals within a culture.	Assures that care will be personalized.
Be sensitive to patients' needs relating to personal space, touching, and religious practices.	Increases patient's sense of acceptance and respect.

ACTIVITIES

Vocabulary Exercise

Complete the puzzle by filling in the missing letters. Use the definitions to help you discover the words.

P

1. _ _ _ _ E _ _ _ _ _ _
2. _ _ _ R _ _ _ _ _ _ _ _
3. _ _ _ _ S
4. _ _ _ _ _ _ O _ _
5. _ _ _ N _ _ _ _ _
6. _ _ A _ _ _ _ _
7. _ _ L _ _ _ _
8. _ _ _ S _ _ _ _ _ _ _
   P
9. _ A _ _
   C
10. _ _ _ _ E _

Definitions

1. Beliefs that are rigid and based on generalizations
2. Feeling of wholeness and connection to the universe and to a power greater than oneself
3. Customs
4. Ritualistic washing
5. Special group within a race as defined by national origin/culture
6. A basis for comparison; a reference point
7. The heritage, traditions, and worldviews of a particular group
8. Ability to be aware of and to appreciate personal characteristics of others
9. Classification of people according to shared physical characteristics
10. Beliefs, views, and morality of a particular group

Short Answer

Briefly answer the following questions.

1. What are the six major ethnic groups in the United States?

   a. _____

   b. _____

   c. _____

   d. _____

   e. _____

   f. _____

2. What effect does living in a new culture have on the cultural values and traditions of the country of origin?

   _____

   _____

   _____

3. People are classified as a race according to which shared physical characteristics?

   _____

   _____

   _____

4. What features do members of ethnic groups have in common?

   _____

   _____

   _____

   _____

   _____

5. What are five cultural differences between ethnic groups?

   a. _____

   b. _____

   c. _____

   d. _____

   e. _____

6. What are three beliefs shared by members of a culture?

   a. _____

   b. _____

   c. _____

True/False

Mark the following true or false by circling T or F.

1. T F Family organization determines who is responsible for health care.

2. T F In Caucasian families, the father is the dominant decision maker.

3. T F In extended families, caregiving and personal care are personal and shared responsibilities.

4. T F A nuclear family usually includes aunts, uncles, and grandparents.

5. T F African Americans prefer to stand far away (more than 3 feet) when speaking with others.

6. T F Asians consider direct eye contact inappropriate.

7. T F Prolonged eye contact is considered disrespectful by Hispanics.

8. T F Shaking hands in Middle Eastern countries is proper only for men.

9. T F In some cultures, the right hand is used for eating and the left hand is used for personal hygiene.

10. T F People who are bilingual may revert to their language of origin when under stress.

RELATING TO THE NURSING PROCESS

Write the step of the nursing process that is related to the nursing assistant action.

Nursing Assistant Action	Nursing Process Step
1. The nursing assistant reports her observations that the patient cannot speak and understand English easily.	_____
2. The nursing assistant stands at a distance that is comfortable for the patient when giving care.	_____
3. The nursing assistant asks politely about practices that are unfamiliar.	_____
4. The nursing assistant provides privacy when a spiritual advisor visits.	_____

DEVELOPING GREATER INSIGHT

1. Your patient, Mr. Dang, is 82 and has lived in this country for several years. He was born in Vietnam, is a Buddhist, and is bilingual.

   a. Of what major ethnic group is Mr. Dang a member?

   _____

   b. What part of his care do you think his family might feel responsible for?

   _____

   c. As a culture, how do Asian Americans feel about direct eye contact?

   _____

   d. Why would it be unwise to stereotype this patient?

   _____

2. Your patient, Ms. Ruiz, is 76. Her leg was fractured in several places when she was hit by a car. She is in balanced traction on your unit. She is originally from Costa Rica and speaks Spanish with limited English. She tells you that her "humours" are out of balance and that she is being punished for past sins. She is a Roman Catholic and wants to see a curandera.

a. How might you improve your ability to communicate with her?

_____

b. What four religious articles might be important to her?

_____

c. In what religious ceremony might she wish to participate?

_____

Infection and Infection Control

Infection

OBJECTIVES

After completing this unit, you will be able to:

- Spell and define terms.
- Identify the most common microbes and describe some of their characteristics.
- List the links in the chain of infection.
- List the ways in which infectious diseases are spread.
- Define spores and explain how spores differ from other pathogens.
- List natural body defenses against infections.
- Explain why patients are at risk for infections.

UNIT SUMMARY

We are surrounded by millions of tiny organisms that cannot be seen with the eye. Like the wind, they make their presence known by their effect, although we cannot see them.

Pathogens are microbes that cause disease. They grow best in a warm, moist, dark environment in which they have a food supply and oxygen needs are met. Infections occur when pathogens invade the body and cause disease.

Pathogens:

- Enter and leave the body by special routes known as *portals of entry* and *portals of exit*
- Transmit disease by direct and indirect means
- May be kept alive in reservoirs

Major types of pathogens include:

- Bacteria

- Viruses

- Fungi

- Protozoa

Protection against infectious disease may be achieved with:

- Natural defenses

- Artificial techniques

Immunization by vaccine to form antibodies against certain infectious diseases is an important form of protection.

Important Types of Pathogens

- Methicillin-resistant *Staphylococcus aureus* (MRSA) and vancomycin-resistant enterococci (VRE) are drug-resistant pathogens that are a major cause of infections acquired in health care facilities.

- Tuberculosis infection occurs when the bacterium enters the body through inhalation. The body creates a barrier that confines the infection. As long as the barrier remains intact, the infection is inactive. Tuberculosis disease develops if the barrier in the lungs breaks down, allowing bacteria to enter the body. This usually occurs as a result of aging or another disease that weakens the immune system.

- *Spores* are microscopic reproductive bodies that are similar to seeds from plants. They are very hardy and difficult to eliminate, and can survive off the body for long periods of time. Spores remain in a dormant form until conditions are ideal for reproduction. When this occurs, they multiply and spread infection. Most infections caused by spores are very serious.

    o Hand hygiene and environmental cleanliness are essential to preventing the spread of spores.

- Shingles (herpes zoster) is a viral infection that occurs in people who were infected by the virus that causes chickenpox. The organisms remain dormant in the body. If the immune system weakens, the organisms become active, causing painful, blister-like lesions on the skin along the paths of sensitive nerves.

- Influenza (flu) is a respiratory infection caused by a family of viruses. Vaccines offer some protection.

- Hepatitis is an inflammation of the liver caused by several viruses:

    o Hepatitis A virus (HAV) is the most common. It is transmitted in feces, saliva, and contaminated food.

    o Hepatitis B virus (HBV) is very serious, and is transmitted by blood, sexual secretions, feces, and saliva. HBV causes liver cancer and death. A vaccine is available to prevent infection.

    o Hepatitis C virus (HCV) is the leading cause of need for liver transplants in the United States. It is spread through blood and body fluid.

    o Other, less common types of hepatitis are hepatitis D, hepatitis E, and hepatitis G. Infection with these organisms is not as serious as the other types.

- Acquired immune deficiency syndrome (AIDS) is a viral disease caused by the human immunodeficiency virus (HIV). It is transmitted through direct contact with the blood and body fluids. Hepatitis B is much more contagious than HIV.

- Severe acute respiratory syndrome (SARS) is a very serious viral respiratory illness that was first seen in China in late 2002. No vaccine is available to prevent infection.

- Your bandage scissors and stethoscope can be fomites if they are not kept very clean. As fomites, these personal items may transfer pathogens from one patient to the next. If personal equipment items will be used during a procedure, wash them with an alcohol product or soap and water before and after each use. If you use a cloth stethoscope tubing cover, wash it each day with your uniform. Carry extra covers so you can change the cover if it becomes contaminated.

NURSING ASSISTANT ALERT

Action	Benefit
Learn the names and characteristics of common microbes.	Achieve better understanding of the nature of germs, disease transmission, and control.
Relate the infection process to the transmission of infection.	Assists in gaining control over disease transmission. Ensures safety of patients and health care providers.
Take appropriate immunizations.	Protects patients and health care providers from infection.

ACTIVITIES

Vocabulary Exercise

Complete the crossword puzzle by using the definitions presented.

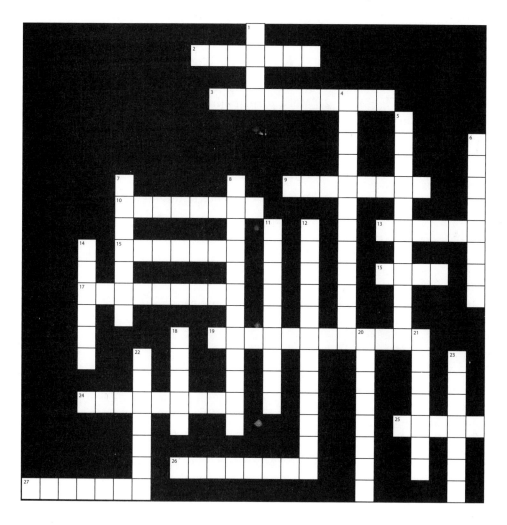

Across

2 Objects containing a pathogen, such as soiled linen

3 A _____ infection develops in a health care facility.

Down

1 Casings for head lice eggs that are firmly attached to the hair shaft

9 Yellow color of the eyes or skin seen in hepatitis and other conditions

10 Simple one-celled microbes that may cause infection in the skin, lungs, urinary tract, and bloodstream

13 Microscopic reproductive bodies that are similar to seeds dispersed from plants

15 An infection may be spread by direct _____ when a person touches another person who is the reservoir of the pathogens.

16 The parasite that causes scabies

17 The place where the pathogen lives and reproduces

19 Dirty or soiled

24 An infection of the liver

25 Microbes that live in and on body surfaces

26 Disease-causing microbe

27 Stealthy, fast moving parasites that usually bite at night when a person is asleep

4 Artificial defense provided by vaccines that protects against a specific pathogen

5 The _____ host is a person who cannot resist a pathogen and will become ill from entry of the pathogen into the body.

6 A _____ lives in or on another organism without benefiting the host.

7 A localized infection, such as a boil

8 The use of biological agents for terrorist purposes

11 The _____ agent is the microbe that causes the infection.

12 The mode of _____ is the method by which infection is spread.

14 A pathogen enters the body through a _____ of entry.

18 If one link of the _____ of infection is broken, the infection will not spread.

20 Substance in the blood that provides immunity (resistance) to infection

21 Moist particles that are spread in the air by people coughing, sneezing, talking, laughing, whistling, spitting, or singing

22 An itchy skin rash caused by a parasite that cannot be seen with the eye

23 Person who is infectious and can give a disease to others

Matching

Match the type of organism to the type of disease or infection it commonly causes.

Disease

1. _____ diarrhea

2. _____ abscess

3. _____ head lice

4. _____ AIDS

5. _____ herpes

6. _____ hepatitis

7. _____ scabies

8. _____ tuberculosis

9. _____ influenza

10. _____ athlete's foot

Organism

a. bacterium

b. virus

c. spores

d. yeast

e. parasite

Completion

Complete the statements in the spaces provided.

1. A human carrier is a person who _____

   _____.

2. The *causative agent* of infectious disease means the _____

   _____.

3. The type (location) of an infection can be:

   a. _____

   b. _____

   c. _____

4. List three ways microbes may be spread.

   a. _____

   b. _____

   c. _____

5. Name the six components of the chain of infection.

   a. _____

   b. _____

   c. _____

   d. _____

   e. _____

   f. _____

6. Three common viruses that cause hepatitis are:

   a. _____

   b. _____

   c. _____

7. Why is hepatitis a major public health concern? _____

   _____

8. What organ is most commonly damaged as a result of hepatitis? _____

   _____

9. Why is proper functioning of this organ so important to overall body function and health? _____

   _____

10. Two groups of organisms that have become resistant to antibiotics are:

    a. methicillin-resistant _____

    b. vancomycin-resistant _____

True/False

Mark the following true or false by circling T or F.

1. T F People who are HIV-positive are less resistant to infection.
2. T F Tuberculosis disease is not infectious.
3. T F Skin testing can identify antibodies to tuberculosis in the body.
4. T F HIV is much more infectious than hepatitis B.
5. T F MRSA is not commonly contracted in health care facilities.
6. T F Infection with certain pathogens causes severe diarrhea.
7. T F Bioterrorism involves the use of biological agents for terrorist purposes.
8. T F Spores cannot spread disease.
9. T F Spores cannot live long in a dormant form.
10. T F Spores are readily eliminated with alcohol and many disinfectants.
11. T F Shingles are not contagious.
12. T F A patient who is jaundiced will have a gray tinge to the skin.
13. T F SARS is caused by a virus.
14. T F Nits are easily removed by brushing them off the hair and scalp.
15. T F The scabies mite is a parasite.
16. T F Scabies is rarely contagious.
17. T F Bedbugs are imaginary pests from a nursery rhyme.
18. T F Dark spots in the bed are a strong indication that bedbugs are present.
19. T F Bedbugs can live for up to a year without food.
20. T F Head lice fly from person to person.

Clinical Situations

1. Your patient, Alan Corbin, is 19 years old and is in end-stage AIDS. Mark the following questions true or false to demonstrate your understanding of the disease.

   a. T F The disease is caused by a bacterium.
   b. T F Everyone who comes in contact with the organism becomes ill with AIDS.
   c. T F HIV destroys the red blood cells.
   d. T F Progression of the disease is determined by the effect of the viruses on the red blood cells.
   e. T F Touching or hugging an AIDS patient will transmit the disease.
   f. T F HIV can be transmitted by contact with blood or contaminated instruments used in medical procedures and tattooing.

2. Mrs. Bustemonte is 67 years of age and a patient on your unit. She has an indwelling catheter. She has a urinary tract infection and urinates frequently. She tells you that she has burning on urination. She also has an elevated temperature (100.8°F). List four actions you should take when caring for her. Choose terms from the list provided.

adequate	back	catheter	empty
front	less	urine	

a. Assist in maintaining _____ fluid levels.

b. Report to the nurse if she eats _____ food.

c. Assist with toileting to keep the bladder _____.

d. Clean the perineal area wiping from _____ to _____.

e. Perform _____ care as directed.

f. Report changes in the character of the _____.

3. Complete the chain of infection.

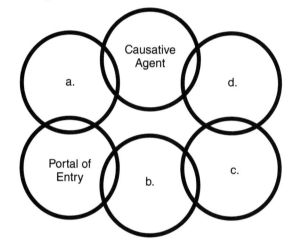

a. _____

b. _____

c. _____

d. _____

4. If one link in the chain of infection is broken, _____

_____.

5. Give five examples of fomites found in the health care facility.

a. _____

b. _____

c. _____

d. _____

e. _____

RELATING TO THE NURSING PROCESS

Nursing Assistant Action	Nursing Process Step
1. The nursing assistant reports an elevation of Mr. Bergen's temperature and redness near his infusion site.	_____
2. The nursing assistant makes sure that Mr. Popejoy, who has pneumonia, has plenty of tissues and a place to dispose of them.	_____
3. The nursing assistant reports that Mr. Menendez was coughing frequently as he was admitted.	_____
4. The nursing assistant collects a urine specimen from Jana Cardillo, a patient in isolation.	_____
5. The nursing assistant attends Chelsea Bolin's care conference.	_____
6. The nursing assistant reports that Mrs. Estes's fever broke when the hypothermia blanket was used.	_____

DEVELOPING GREATER INSIGHT

Match the action with the related portion of the chain of infection.

1. _____ Receiving antibiotics when infected

2. _____ Disinfecting bedpans

3. _____ Covering a draining pressure ulcer

4. _____ Not coming to work when you have a cold

5. _____ Putting a plastic bandage strip over a cut in your skin

a. protecting the portal of entry

b. protecting the portal of exit

c. protecting a susceptible host

d. controlling the causative agents

e. eliminating the reservoir

Infection Control

OBJECTIVES

After completing this unit, you will be able to:

- Spell and define terms.
- Explain the principles of medical asepsis.
- Explain the components of standard precautions.
- Describe nursing assistant actions related to standard precautions.
- Describe airborne, droplet, and contact precautions.
- List the types of personal protective equipment and discuss the use of each item.
- Demonstrate Procedures 1–7 (set out in this unit in the textbook).

UNIT SUMMARY

When patients have communicable diseases that are easily transmitted to others, special techniques must be used. Such a patient is placed in isolation. Everyone who comes into contact with the patient must practice appropriate isolation techniques. The emphasis is on the infectious material that carries the specific microorganisms. The goal of the health care provider is to interrupt the chain of infection by preventing transmission of the microbes. By working toward this goal, the health care provider protects the patient, the environment, and self.

The spread of disease can be controlled by:

- Conscientious handwashing
- Proper medical and surgical asepsis
- Understanding and faithfully following:
  - Standard precautions
  - Transmission-based precautions
  - Isolation techniques
  - Disinfection and sterilization procedures

NURSING ASSISTANT ALERT

Action	Benefit
Follow standard precautions exactly.	Prevents transfer of infectious materials.
Give extra attention to isolation patients.	Prevents patient from feeling abandoned.
Place sharps in proper container.	Decreases the danger of needle or sharp sticks.
Follow specific transmission-based precautions as outlined in care plan.	Eliminates unnecessary actions while ensuring that specific transmission prevention techniques are used.
Follow aseptic techniques carefully and accurately.	Protects patients and health care providers from infection.

ACTIVITIES

Vocabulary Exercise

Put a circle around each word defined. Use the terms in the list provided.

CDC	communicable	dirty	disposable	droplet
feces	gloves	goggles	gown	HEPA
HIV	isolate	negative	standard	

e	o	P	Q	e	v	i	t	a	g	e	n
s	l	s	h	s	e	l	g	g	o	g	d
t	d	b	e	V	S	d	w	M	C	i	e
a	r	k	a	c	l	E	j	D	r	l	h
n	o	s	v	c	e	H	C	t	b	G	L
d	p	e	E	M	i	f	y	a	Z	a	F
a	l	v	g	C	M	n	s	W	o	V	M
r	e	o	R	o	g	o	u	A	u	C	M
d	t	l	e	o	p	m	h	m	P	C	w
j	x	g	w	s	C	n	W	G	m	E	d
t	A	n	i	l	a	W	k	K	J	o	H
c	C	d	i	s	o	l	a	t	e	g	c

1. spreads long distances in the air on dust and moisture

2. Centers for Disease Control and Prevention

3. an infectious disease easily transmitted to others

4. protective hand coverings

5. expendable

6. separate ill patients from others

7. waste products of the body

8. eye protection that is always worn with a mask

9. one type of mask used in airborne precautions

10. human immunodeficiency virus

11. Air flow in an airborne precautions room is reversed, creating a _____-pressure environment.

12. unclean

13. _____ precautions are used any time contact with blood, body fluid, secretions, excretions, mucous membranes, or nonintact skin is likely.

14. PPE that covers the uniform

True/False

Mark the following true or false by circling T or F.

1. T F Linen found on a linen cart is considered clean.

2. T F Linen that has touched the floor is clean as long as the floor is not wet.

3. T F Medical aseptic techniques destroy all organisms on an article.

4. T F One patient's articles may be used by another as long as the first patient does not have a communicable disease.

When washing hands correctly:

5. T F Always use cool water.

6. T F Lean against the sink so no water will get on the floor.

7. T F A soap dispenser is preferable to a bar of soap.

8. T F You need not wash your hands if they are not visibly soiled.

9. T F Turn faucets on and off with gloves.

10. T F Always point fingertips up when washing.

11. T F It is the use of soap that actually removes microbes from hands.

12. T F Hands can be washed effectively in 5 to 10 seconds.

13. T F Personal medical asepsis includes a daily bath.

14. T F Complete personal protective equipment is required for all work with patients.

15. T F Alcohol gel may be used instead of handwashing, unless the hands are visibly soiled.

16. T F When using an alcohol-based hand cleaner, rub the product into all surfaces for at least 15 seconds.

17. T F Handwashing is not necessary if gloves were worn during patient care.

18. T F You can safely touch environmental surfaces with used gloves as long as the gloves are not contaminated with blood.

19. T F The nursing assistant is responsible for understanding the principles of standard precautions and selecting personal protective equipment appropriate to the procedure.

20. T F Wash your gloves promptly if they become soiled.

21. T F Artificial nails are usually acceptable for health care workers as long as the nails have been professionally applied.

22. T F The housekeeping cart and the clean linen cart should be positioned close to each other in the hallway.

Completion

Complete the statements in the spaces provided.

1. The purpose of transmission-based precautions is _____
   _____.

2. When working in droplet precautions, you would wear a mask when you work within _____
   feet of the patient.

3. Isolation is the responsibility of _____.

4. The purpose of wearing a mask and gown in the isolation unit is to _____
   _____.

5. Gloves should be used whenever there may be contact with _____
   _____.

6. To be effective, a mask must cover both _____.

7. To be effective, a gown should _____ correctly.

8. The contaminated gown should be folded _____ before you dispose of it in the proper
   receptacle.

9. Disposable equipment is used only _____.

10. List four secretions or excretions that are potentially infectious.

    a._____

    b._____

    c._____

    d._____

11. Breaks in the skin of a health care worker should be immediately treated by _____ and
    applying _____.

12. What do these six items have in common before they are used?

    stethoscope   glass thermometer   bathtub

    shower chair   tympanic thermometer   wheelchair

    _____

    _____

Short Answer

1. Name the type of infection control that is used in all situations in which care providers may contact body
   fluids. _____

2. List the three types of transmission-based precautions.

   a. _____

   b. _____

   c. _____

3. List three ways communicable diseases may be spread.

a. _____

b. _____

c. _____

4. List six articles to be placed on a cart outside an isolation room (or in the anteroom).

a. _____

b. _____

c. _____

d. _____

e. _____

f. _____

5. State the sequence for applying personal protective equipment.

a. _____

b. _____

c. _____

d. _____

6. List four precautions to keep in mind when handling soiled linen.

a. _____

b. _____

c. _____

d. _____

7. State the measures that are to be taken to care for vital sign equipment used with a patient in isolation.

a. _____

b. _____

8. Name the type of bag that is used for the transport of specimens. _____

9. Name two ways to sterilize an item.

a. _____

b. _____

10. List three respiratory hygiene/cough etiquette practices that patients should be instructed to follow to prevent the spread of infection.

a. _____

b. _____

c. _____

11. UVGI

    a. uses _____ light in the _____ or _____ .

    b. The purpose of UVGI is to _____ .

    c. Does the UVGI light remain on 24 hours a day? _____

    d. Does the radiation emitted from the bright UVGI harm patients' or staff members' eyes? _____

    _____

12. When entering the room of a patient who is in contact precautions, what PPE should you apply?

    _____

    _____

13. When working within 3 feet of a patient with a droplet infection, you should apply_____

    _____

    _____

14. In addition to UVGI lighting, is a negative pressure environment also necessary for tuberculosis isolation?

    _____

    _____

15. When leaving the airborne precautions room, where is PPE removed?

    _____

    _____

16. Where should the respirator be removed when you have finished working in the airborne precautions room?

    _____

    _____

17. Can the face mask be reused during your shift when caring for a patient in droplet precautions?

    _____

    _____

Clinical Situations

Briefly describe how a nursing assistant should react to the following situations.

1. You saw an airborne precautions sign on Mr. Keene's door. You must serve his breakfast tray.

    _____

    _____

    _____

2. You are responsible for caring for nondisposable equipment from a contact precautions unit.

    _____

    _____

Identification

1. Identify the sign and indicate the type of precaution to be used.

a.

_____

_____

b.

_____

_____

c.

_____

_____

d.

_____

_____

e.

_____

_____

2. Label the diagram of the isolation room.

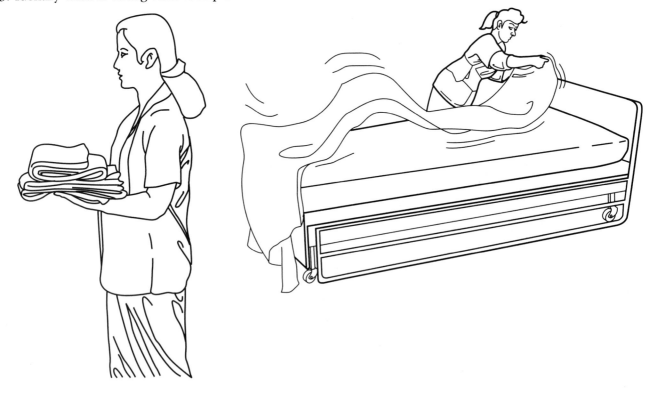

a. _____

b. _____

c. _____

3. Identify what is wrong with each picture. What should be done to correct it?

a. Error _____   c. Error _____

b. Correction _____   d. Correction _____

4. What is wrong with the figure on the left? Correct it in the figure on the right. Use the empty bedside table to demonstrate the correction by drawing in the articles or writing the names of the articles.

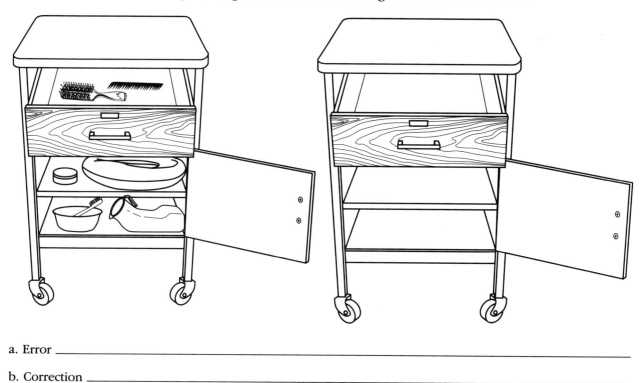

a. Error _____

b. Correction _____

RELATING TO THE NURSING PROCESS

Write the step of the nursing process that is related to the nursing assistant action.

Nursing Assistant Action	Nursing Process Step

1. The nursing assistant is not sure about how to transport the patient safely from isolation to the X-ray department, so she asks the team leader for instructions. _____

2. The nursing assistant carefully removes his contaminated gown and disposes of it properly after completing care in the contact precautions room. _____

3. Mr. DeLong had a fever at 8:00. The nursing assistant rechecks his temperature at 11:00. _____

4. The nursing assistant reviews the care plan for Mrs. Bruckner, who is in contact precautions. The assistant organizes her assignment to allow enough time to meet patient needs. The assistant determines which supplies will be needed in the isolation room. _____

5. The nursing assistant readjusts her priorities and cares for other patients when Mrs. Bruckner has an unexpected visitor. _____

6. The nursing assistant learns a new approach to a procedure in a staff development class. She uses the procedure in Mrs. Bruckner's care and discusses its effectiveness with the nurse. _____

7. The nursing assistant follows the restorative approaches on Mrs. Bruckner's care plan and compliments the patient on improving her self-care ability. _____

8. The nursing assistant obtains the admission height and weight for a patient who was admitted to an airborne precautions room. _____

DEVELOPING GREATER INSIGHT

1. Mrs. Bruckner says she is tired of drinking "hot water," and asks the nursing assistant to fill her water pitcher with ice. Can the assistant fill the water pitcher at the ice machine in the unit's pantry?

_____

_____

2. What is the best method of ensuring that Mrs. Bruckner gets a pitcher full of fresh ice without risking contamination of others on the unit?

_____

_____

3. The nursing assistant returns to Mrs. Bruckner's room with fresh ice for the water pitcher, which is on the overbed table next to the bed. She plans to put fresh water in the pitcher using the sink in the room. What PPE will she apply when entering the room?

_____

_____

4. The laboratory reports have just been sent to the unit. The stool culture reveals that Mrs. Bruckner has diarrhea caused by *Clostridium difficile*, a spore-producing pathogen. After finishing patient care and removing PPE, describe what the assistant must do before leaving the room.

_____

_____

Safety and Mobility

Environmental and Nursing Assistant Safety

OBJECTIVES

After completing this unit, you will be able to:

- Spell and define terms.
- Describe the health care facility environment.
- Identify measures to promote environmental safety.
- Describe the elements required for a fire.
- List five measures to prevent fires.
- Describe the procedure to follow if a fire occurs.
- Describe the PASS procedure.
- List at least 10 guidelines for dealing with a violent individual.
- List techniques for using ergonomics on the job.
- Demonstrate appropriate body mechanics.
- Describe the types of information contained in Material Safety Data Sheets.

UNIT SUMMARY

The nursing staff is responsible for maintaining a safe, comfortable environment for the patient.

- The bed and unit are the patient's home during the stay at the facility.

- All equipment must be readily available and kept in clean operating condition.

- Safety is the business of everyone. Knowing the rules ensures your full participation.

- The cleanliness of the unit must be maintained on a daily basis. The unit must be completely cleaned before being used by a new patient.

- Fire is a potential threat. All staff must be aware of potential fire hazards and control them. Facility emergency plans and procedures must be understood and followed in case of a fire.

- Knowledge of ergonomics can prevent worker injuries.

- Knowledge of chemicals used is required by federal law.

NURSING ASSISTANT ALERT

Action	Benefit
Maintain an even temperature, regulating light and ventilation.	Contributes to patient comfort.
Report equipment in need of repair.	Prevents possible accidents and injury.
Use proper body mechanics.	Avoids injury to patient and caregiver.
Apply restraints and supports according to established protocol.	Ensures proper standard of patient care.
Know and follow fire safety policies.	Ensures patients and staff greatest opportunities for safe exit during a fire emergency.

ACTIVITIES

Vocabulary Exercise

Each line has four different spellings of a word from this unit. Circle the correctly spelled word.

1. incident	incedent	incidant	incydent
2. ralys	rails	riles	rhales
3. warde	werd	ward	whard
4. privite	privat	pryvate	private
5. ergonomecs	ergonomics	erkonomics	ergonomicks
6. concurent	concurrent	concurrant	concarrent
7. seme private	semiprivote	semepryvate	semiprivate
8. envyromental	environmantyl	environmental	enviromental

Completion

Complete the statements related to safety practices by writing the correct term from the list provided in the blank spaces.

alcohol	all health care	within reach	calm
checked	concern	electrical	fuel
grounded	hazard	heat	incident
instrument	locked	MSDS	nail polish remover
never	nurse	oils	OSHA
oxygen	patients	right away	
supervisor	shut off	tagged	
work	work-related	72	

1. Keeping the environment safe and clean is the responsibility of _____ workers.

2. Prevention of injuries to patients and others is of primary _____.

3. Wheels should always be _____ unless a bed is being moved.

4. The best temperature for the patient's room is about _____ degrees.

5. When leaving the patient's room, be sure that the ceiling lights are _____.

6. Frayed _____ cords should be reported at once.

7. For safety, use an _____ to pick up broken glass.

8. An unexpected, undesirable event that occurs in a health care facility is called a/an _____.

9. When equipment is broken, it is _____.

10. Mechanical lifts should be _____ before use.

11. Plugs that are not properly _____ are a fire hazard.

12. Smoking in bed should _____ be permitted.

13. Make sure call signal controls are always _____.

14. The three elements that form the fire triangle are _____, _____, and _____.

15. Possible fire hazards should be reported _____ to the _____.

16. When oxygen is in use, flammable liquids such as _____, _____, or _____ should not be used.

17. When there is an emergency, it is very important for you to keep _____.

18. When there is a fire, always move _____ to safety first.

19. The term *ergonomic* refers to _____ musculoskeletal conditions.

20. The federal agency that is responsible for employee safety is called _____.

21. Hazards communication information called _____ must be supplied by manufacturers, by law.

Short Answer

Write the information in the spaces provided.

1. Briefly list nine components of the patient's environment.

   a. _____

   b. _____

   c. _____

   d. _____

   e. _____

   f. _____

   g. _____

   h. _____

   i. _____

2. Name two pieces of fire control equipment.

   a. _____

   b. _____

3. The acronym PASS is important for fire control. The

   a. P stands for _____.

   b. A stands for _____.

   c. S stands for _____.

   d. S stands for _____.

4. List six ergonomic techniques you can use to decrease the risk of injury.

   a. _____

   b. _____

   c. _____

   d. _____

   e. _____

   f. _____

5. State three types of information you expect to learn from the MSDS of a product.

   a. _____

   b. _____

   c. _____

6. List six potential ways of preventing violence in the health care facility.

   a. _____

   b. _____

   c. _____

   d. _____

   e. _____

   f. _____

7. List six methods of dealing with a violent individual.

a. _____

b. _____

c. _____

d. _____

e. _____

f. _____

8. Draw the fire triangle, showing its elements.

Hidden Picture

Look carefully at the picture and list each violation of a safety measure in the spaces provided.

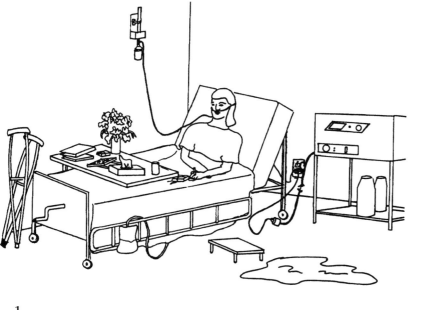

1. _____

2. _____

3. _____

4. _____

5. _____

6. _____

7. _____

8. _____

9. _____

10. _____

11. _____

12. _____

13. _____

RELATING TO THE NURSING PROCESS

Write the step of the nursing process that is related to the nursing assistant action.

Nursing Assistant Action	**Nursing Process Step**
1. The nursing assistant participates in a conference regarding patient evacuation in case of an emergency.	_____
2. The nursing team, including the nursing assistants, participates in a training session to prepare for actions to take if a patient experiences a cardiac arrest.	_____
3. The nursing assistant checks the setting on the oxygen each time he is in the room.	_____
4. The nursing assistant follows the care plan and uses the mechanical lift to move the patient.	_____
5. The nursing assistant closely observes the stroke patient's ability to use the right hand and reports the findings to the nurse.	_____
6. The patient refuses range of motion, so the nursing assistant discusses methods of ensuring that the patient exercises the joints during activities of daily living.	_____
7. The nurse discusses the use of exercises to maintain range of motion with the nursing assistant. Together they measure the degree of movement in the patient's joints to determine whether joint exercises have been effective in preventing contractures.	_____

DEVELOPING GREATER INSIGHT

1. The liquid oxygen canister in Mr. Heaney's room is hissing when you enter the room to answer the call signal. What is the first action to take?

    a. turn off the call signal.

    b. call for help.

    _____

2. State two reasons for your action in item 1.

    a. _____

    b. _____

3. You will

    a. grab the canister and run outside.

    b. remove the patient from the room.

    _____

4. State the reason for your action in item 3.

    _____

    _____

5. You will

    a. close the door to the room.

    b. pull the fire alarm.

6. State the reason for your action in item 5.

    _____

    _____

Patient Safety and Positioning

OBJECTIVES

After completing this unit, you will be able to:

- Spell and define terms.
- Identify patients who are at risk for having incidents.
- List alternatives to the use of physical restraints.
- Describe the guidelines for the use of restraints.
- Demonstrate the correct application of restraints.
- List the elements that are common to all procedures.
- Describe correct body alignment for the patient.
- List the purposes of repositioning patients.
- Demonstrate these positions using the correct supportive devices: supine, semisupine, prone, semiprone, lateral, Fowler's, and orthopneic.
- Demonstrate Procedures 10–13 (set out in this unit in the textbook).

UNIT SUMMARY

- Preventive measures must be implemented to avoid patient incidents.
- *Enablers* are devices that empower patients and assist patients to function at their highest possible level.
- Alternatives to restraints should be used whenever possible. If restraints are necessary, the least amount of restraint should be used for the least amount of time necessary to keep the patient safe.

- Before restraints are used, the staff must assess the patient's capabilities and reasons for use of the restraint. Eliminating the cause of a problem may eliminate the need for the restraint.
- Restraints, if necessary, must be applied correctly. The care plan and all policies on restraint use must be followed.
- Side rails are restraints in some circumstances. They are also enablers in some situations.

- Care must be taken to keep the patient in good alignment and provide support at all times in all positions.

- Frequent change of position helps prevent deformities and pressure ulcers. It also aids general body function and contributes to comfort.

- Frequent position changes are essential to prevent:

  ○ Musculoskeletal deformities and loss of calcium from bone

  ○ Poor skin nutrition and the development of pressure ulcers

  ○ Respiratory complications such as pneumonia

  ○ Decreased circulation that could lead to thrombophlebitis and renal calculi

  ○ Loss of opportunities for social exchange between patient and staff

- Your bandage scissors, stethoscope, and other personal items may transfer pathogens from one patient to the next. If personal equipment items will be used during a procedure, wash them with an alcohol product or soap and water before and after each use.

Procedures are step-by-step directions for giving patient care. They must be followed faithfully. Some steps are common to all procedures. The initial procedure actions and ending procedure actions are as follows.

Initial Procedure Actions

1. Wash your hands or use an alcohol-based hand cleaner.

2. Assemble supplies and equipment and bring to the patient's room.

3. Knock on the door and identify yourself.

4. Identify the patient according to facility policy.

5. Ask visitors to leave the room and advise where they may wait (as desired by patient).

6. Explain what you are going to do and what is expected of the patient. Answer questions. (Maintain a dialogue with the patient during the procedure and repeat explanations and instructions as needed.)

7. Provide privacy by closing the door, privacy curtain, and window curtain. (All three should be closed even if the patient is alone in the room.)

8. Wash your hands or use an alcohol-based hand cleaner.

9. Set up supplies and equipment at the bedside. (Use an overbed table, if possible, or other clean area. Cover with a clean underpad, according to nursing judgment, to provide a clean work surface.) Open packages. Position items for convenient reach. Position a container for soiled items so that you do not have to cross over clean items to access it.

10. Raise the bed to a comfortable working height.

11. Position the patient for the procedure. Support with pillows and props as needed. Place a clean underpad under the area, as needed. Make sure the patient is comfortable and can maintain the position for the duration of the procedure.

12. Cover the patient with a bath blanket and drape for modesty. Fold the bath blanket back to expose only the area on which you will be working. (This step is essential even if the door, window, and cubicle curtains are closed.)

13. Apply gloves if contact with blood, moist body fluids (except sweat), secretions, excretions, or nonintact skin is likely.

14. Apply a gown if your uniform will have substantial contact with linen or other articles contaminated with blood, moist body fluids (except sweat), secretions, or excretions.

15. Apply a mask and eye protection if splashing of blood or moist body fluids is likely.

16. Lower the side rail on the side where you will be working.

Ending Procedure Actions

1. Remove gloves.

2. Reposition the patient to ensure that he or she is comfortable and in good body alignment.

3. Replace the bed covers, then remove any drapes used. Place used drapes in plastic bag to discard in trash or soiled linen.

4. Elevate the side rails, if used, before leaving the bedside.

5. Remove other personal protective equipment, if worn, and discard in plastic bag or according to facility policy.

6. Wash your hands or use an alcohol-based hand cleaner.

7. Return the bed to the lowest horizontal position.

8. Open the privacy and window curtains.

9. Position the call signal and needed personal items within reach.

10. Wash your hands or use an alcohol-based hand cleaner.

11. Perform a general safety check of the patient and environment.

12. Remove procedural trash and contaminated linen when you leave the room. Discard in appropriate container or location, according to facility policy.

13. Inform visitors that they may return to the room.

14. Document the procedure, your observations, and the patient's response.

Note: When there are open lesions, wet linen, or possible contact with patient body fluids, blood, secretions, excretions, mucous membranes, or non-intact skin, disposable gloves are to be worn during the procedure. Put on gloves before contact with the patient or linen. Dispose of gloves according to facility policy after removing them. *Always apply standard precautions*.

Special procedures in this unit relate to positioning, supporting, and restraining patients in a safe, appropriate manner, using proper body mechanics.

NURSING ASSISTANT ALERT

Action	Benefit
Use proper posture and body mechanics during all activities.	Enables the body to function at its best.
Follow the eight basic rules for effective body use.	Prevents injury and reduces fatigue.
Support patients in proper alignment in all positions.	Improves comfort and relieves strain.
	Prevents deformities.
	Allows the body to function more effectively.
Apply restraints and supports according to established protocol.	Ensures proper standard of patient care.

ACTIVITIES

Vocabulary Exercise

Complete the puzzle by filling in the missing letters of words found in this unit. Use the definitions to help you discover these words.

1. __ P __ __ __ __   1. Involving muscle contractions

2. __ __ __ __ O __ __ __   2. Devices for maintaining the position of extremities

3. __ __ S __ __ __ __ __   3. Device that inhibits patient movement

4. __ __ __ __ I __ __   4. Ability to move

5. __ __ __ T __ __ __ __ __ __   5. Occurs when muscles become fixed in one position

6. __ __ __ I __ __   6. On the back

7. __ __ O __ __ __ __ __   7. Steps to follow to carry out a task

8. __ __ __ __ N __   8. Another term for orthosis

Completion

Complete the statements in the spaces provided.

1. Before beginning any patient contact, you must _____ and _____.

2. A good principle to follow is never to attempt to move a patient who weighs more than you do if you are _____.

3. A heavy or helpless patient can be more easily positioned in bed if a _____ is used.

4. A good way to help a patient maintain a side-lying position is to form a pillow roll and place it

   _____

   _____.

5. Before rolling a patient away from you, be sure the _____

   _____.

6. When moving a patient to the head of the bed, the nursing assistant should _____ the head of the bed.

7. The patient's position must be changed at least every _____.

8. In the prone position, the bed is in the _____ position and the patient is placed on his _____.

9. Two forms of restraint are _____ and _____.

10. When restraints are released, the patient must be _____.

11. Three incidents that may occur are _____, _____, and _____ injury.

True/False

Mark the following true or false by circling T or F.

1. T F Restraints should be used only as a last resort.

2. T F Side rails may safely be left down when restraints are in use.

3. T F Restraints should be secured to the immovable part of the bed frame.

4. T F To prevent accidental poisoning, store a patient's personal food items in the bedside table.

5. T F When preparing bath water, always turn the hot water on last.

6. T F Using a microwave oven to reheat foods is safe and economical because food is evenly heated.

7. T F Always knock before entering a room.

8. T F Special boots or shoes may be worn in bed to maintain feet in the proper alignment.

9. T F A patient positioned on her left side should be moved to the left side of the bed.

10. T F A trochanter roll should extend from under the arm, along the trunk, to the top of the hip.

Short Answer

Briefly explain the reasoning behind each of the following statements.

1. The nursing assistant should use leg muscles and shoulder muscles to lift and not the muscles of the back. Why?

   _____

   _____

2. Proper positioning of the patient's body must be conscientiously done because

_____

_____

_____

3. The staff must take specific steps before applying restraints. What are these steps and why must they be done?

_____

_____

Name the Position

In the space provided on the left, name the position pictured on the right.

1. _____

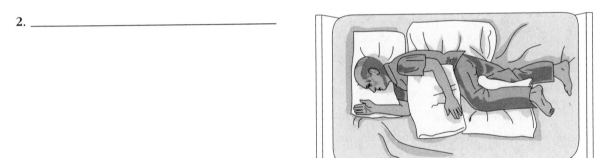

2. _____

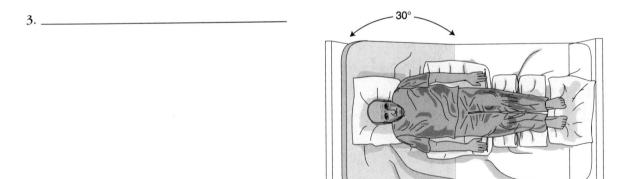

3. _____

Clinical Situations

1. Mrs. Grover wears a hearing aid and glasses. She has difficulty ambulating and is unsteady on her feet. She is sometimes disoriented and tends to wander when she becomes hungry, in search of food. List ways a nursing assistant might protect this patient and avoid the need for protective restraints.

   a. _____

   b. _____

   c. _____

   d. _____

   e. _____

   f. _____

2. What physical restraints might be used if alternatives fail and the protocol for restraints has been followed?

   a. _____

   b. _____

   c. _____

   d. _____

   e. _____

3. Mr. Kinsey is 82 years of age, weighs 215 pounds, and has a respiratory problem (emphysema). He tends to slide to the foot of the bed and has difficulty staying comfortable. What actions should you take when you find him in this position?

   a. _____

   b. _____

   c. _____

RELATING TO THE NURSING PROCESS

Write the step of the nursing process that is related to the nursing assistant action.

Nursing Assistant Action	Nursing Process Step
1. The nursing assistant applies a restraint alternative that is listed on the care plan. He informs the nurse that the patient's agitation decreased when the restraint was removed and the alternative was used.	_____
2. The care plan states to turn Mr. Bernardi *"every two hours or more often, as needed."* You plan to turn him at least every 90 minutes because his skin is beginning to break down.	_____
3. You follow the care plan and position Mr. Bernardi in the 90-90-90 position when he is sitting up in the wheelchair.	_____
4. To maintain Mr. Bernardi in good sitting alignment, you add a foam roll to the right side of the wheelchair.	_____
5. You notify the nurse that Mr. Bernardi looked good when he was sitting in the 90-90-90 position in the wheelchair, and thanked you for positioning him so comfortably.	_____
6. The nurse asked you to weigh Mr. Bernardi, then check the restraint chart to identify the correct size vest so she could write it on the care plan.	_____

DEVELOPING GREATER INSIGHT

You were picking up lunch trays and found Mr. Bernardi choking on his food. You yelled out for help, but no one has responded yet. The patient is becoming cyanotic, cannot speak, and looks terrified. You recognize that you must free the obstruction in his airway. However, Mr. Bernardi is wearing a vest restraint and someone has tied it tightly in a knot that you cannot undo. The restraint is too tight to remove or pull over the patient's head.

1. What action should you take?

   _____

2. Why?

   _____

The Patient's Mobility: Transfer Skills

OBJECTIVES

After completing this unit, you will be able to:

- Spell and define terms.

- Apply the principles of good body mechanics and ergonomics to moving and transferring patients.

- Describe the difference between a standing transfer and a sitting transfer.

- List at least seven factors to consider before moving a patient, to determine whether additional equipment or assistance is necessary.

- List the guidelines for safe transfers.

- Demonstrate correct application of a transfer belt.

- Demonstrate Procedures 14–21 (set out in this unit in the textbook).

UNIT SUMMARY

Assisting patients to make transfers safely is an important nursing assistant function. There are basically two types of transfers:

1. Sitting transfers

2. Standing transfers

The type of transfer ordered depends on the patient's:

- Strength, endurance, and balance

- Mental condition

- Size

Equipment used to facilitate transfers includes:

- Transfer belts

- Mechanical lifts

- Sliding boards

Transfers must be carried out smoothly, using proper body mechanics, to assure comfort and safety for both patient and worker.

- In a standing transfer, the patient stands during the transfer.

- In a sitting transfer, the patient sits throughout the transfer, such as when a mechanical lift is used.

- A lateral transfer involves moving a sitting patient to the side, such as when a sliding board is used.

Nursing work is one of the top 10 occupations for work-related musculoskeletal injuries. Having a previous history of back injury is the greatest risk factor for a new back injury or back pain. Workers with a history of injury have twice as many injuries compared with workers who have no history of back problems.

Moving patients is the task with the highest risk of injury because workers do not use their bodies or equipment correctly, or end up in awkward positions and confined spaces, where they must bend or reach while the back is flexed.

Having a "no-lift" policy does not mean that workers should never lift a patient, heavy box, or equipment. Instead, it means that no manual lifting should be done. Remember, your back must last a lifetime. You must adapt the procedures in your book to the policies, procedures, and equipment available in your facility for moving patients and protecting your back.

NURSING ASSISTANT ALERT

Action	Benefit
Check equipment before using.	Unsafe equipment can be replaced and injury avoided.
Be sure bed and wheelchair or stretcher are locked before transfer.	Prevents potential accidents, injury, and deformity.
Explain procedure before transfer.	Enables patient to assist if possible.
Evaluate situation and get help if needed.	Reduces patient fears. Avoids injury to patient and staff.
Use proper transfer techniques.	Avoids injury to patient and caregivers.

ACTIVITIES

Vocabulary Exercise

Complete each sentence using the best term from the list provided.

dependent	full weight	gait	paralyzed
partial weight	pivot	self	sitting

1. A mechanical lift may be used to transfer a _____ patient.

2. Having the ability to stand on both legs is called _____ bearing.

3. The ability to stand on one leg is called _____ bearing.

4. A _____ patient does not have the ability to move.

5. A transfer belt is also called a _____ belt.

6. To _____ means to rotate the entire body to one side.

Completion

Complete the statements in the spaces provided.

1. Before attempting to move a patient, always determine if _____ is needed.

2. Before transferring a patient from bed to chair, you should know whether the patient is _____- bearing.

3. When assisting a patient from bed to wheelchair, make sure that the wheelchair footrests are _____.

4. When moving a patient with a mechanical lift, make sure the sling is positioned from _____ to _____.

5. Four people should be positioned to move an unconscious person from a stretcher to bed, as follows:

_____

_____

_____

_____

Corrections

Correct the statements that are wrong by crossing out the incorrect word or words. Write the correct words under them. Do not make any changes in the correct statements.

1. Know a patient's capabilities before attempting a transfer.

2. Allow patients to place their hands around your neck.

3. Use a lift sheet for standing transfers.

4. Always explain the transfer plan to the patient.

5. Transfer patients toward their weakest side.

6. Patient shoes should have smooth soles and heels if the facility has tile floors.

7. Placing your hands under the patient's arms is acceptable during transfers.

8. IVs, drainage bags, and other items must be considered during a transfer.

9. Give the patient who is transferring only the assistance he needs.

10. Before making a transfer, put the bed in the high horizontal position.

11. Always use correct body mechanics when making transfers.

_____

12. During transfer, encourage the patient to focus her eyes on your hands.

_____

13. Stand close to the patient during a transfer.

_____

True/False

Mark the following true or false by circling T or F.

1. T F A transfer belt is used to assist patients to transfer.
2. T F A transfer belt can be used to lift a patient who has no ability to bear weight.
3. T F A transfer belt should be applied under the patient's clothing.
4. T F Always apply a transfer belt with the patient lying on her side.
5. T F The buckle of the transfer belt should be positioned in the front.
6. T F The transfer belt should be positioned around a female patient's breasts.
7. T F The transfer belt should be held using an underhand grasp.
8. T F The use of a transfer belt is contraindicated for a patient with abdominal aneurysm.
9. T F The transfer belt can be removed after the transfer is complete.
10. T F The transfer belt should be very tight.

Clinical Situations

Briefly describe how a nursing assistant should react in the following situations.

1. No one is available in the radiology department when you arrive. You need help to move a patient.

_____

2. Your heavy patient is unable to help himself. He has returned from physical therapy and needs to be returned to bed.

_____

3. You must assist one other person to transfer a conscious patient from a stretcher to bed following an X-ray.

_____

_____

4. You are assigned to transfer a patient to a chair using a mechanical lift. The sling is frayed where it hooks onto the lift frame.

_____

_____

5. Mr. Dunn is able to be up but is unstable when standing. He needs to empty his bladder.

_____

_____

Identification

Look carefully at each picture. List the corrections that should be made in each.

1.

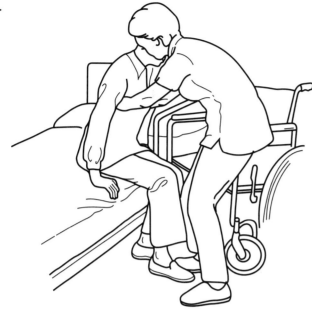

Corrections

a. _____

b. _____

c. _____

2.

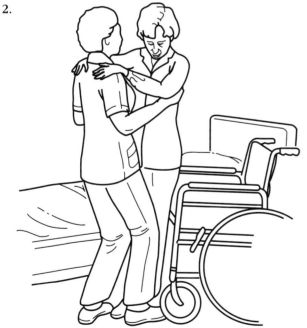

Corrections

a. _____

b. _____

c. _____

3.

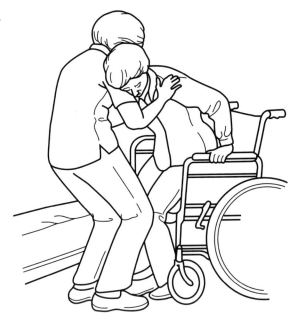

Corrections

a. _____

b. _____

c. _____

4.

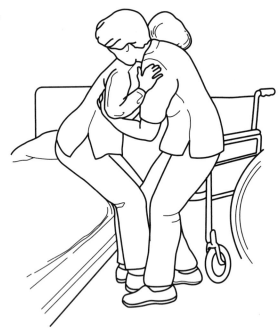

Corrections

a. _____

b. _____

c. _____

RELATING TO THE NURSING PROCESS

Write the step of the nursing process that is related to the nursing assistant action.

Nursing Assistant Action

1. The nursing assistant carefully applies the transfer belt.

2. The nursing assistant reports that the patient weighs 216 pounds and is paralyzed on the right side.

3. The nursing assistant assembles all needed equipment at the bedside before attempting a transfer.

4. The nursing assistant carefully checks the mechanical lift before using it.

5. The nursing assistant informs the nurse that the patient's ability to transfer has improved, and she is now able to walk to the bathroom with the walker and a standby assist. Last week the patient required 2 assistants to transfer, and could take only a few steps.

6. The nursing assistant attends care conference and provides information that is added to the care plan.

Nursing Process Step

_____

_____

_____

_____

_____

_____

DEVELOPING GREATER INSIGHT

Answer the questions below based on the following situation.

You are assigned to transfer Mr. Youngren from bed to chair and back. The care plan states that you are to use a one-person assist, using a transfer belt, for this patient. The patient's daughter arrives to visit when you are preparing to transfer the patient to the chair. She insists that you remove the transfer belt, and tells you to lift the patient by grabbing him under the arms like she does at home. She says she does not trust that fabric belt and insists that her father will fall if it is used. You have transferred Mr. Youngren with the belt before and had no problems. Before you have a chance to respond, she grabs her father under the arms and moves him to the chair. She tells you to use this method next time you move him.

1. How will you respond to the patient's daughter?

_____

2. Will you use the transfer belt to transfer Mr. Youngren in the future?

_____

3. Is it necessary to report this situation to the nurse?

_____

4. Explain your answer to number 3.

_____

The Patient's Mobility: Ambulation

OBJECTIVES

After completing this unit, you will be able to:

- Spell and define terms.
- State the purpose of assistive devices used in ambulation.
- List safety measures for using assistive devices.
- Describe safety measures for using a wheelchair.
- Describe nursing assistant actions for:
  - Ambulating a patient using a gait belt.
  - Propelling a patient in a wheelchair.
  - Positioning a patient in a wheelchair.
  - Transporting a patient on a stretcher.
- Demonstrate Procedures 22–24 (set out in this unit in the textbook).

UNIT SUMMARY

Nursing assistants frequently assist patients with ambulation. Ambulating with assistance may require the use of an assistive device. Such assistive devices include:

- Gait belt
- Walkers
- Crutches
- Canes

Nursing assistants must be competent in applying and using assistive devices safely.

- Patients must be positioned correctly in wheelchairs, with props used as needed to keep the patient in good alignment.
- The wheelchair must fit the patient correctly.
- Pressure ulcers can develop when a patient is sitting in a wheelchair. Pay attention to pressure relief when the patient is seated.

- Patients are also transported in wheelchairs and stretchers, and correct techniques and safety measures must be applied for vehicle use.

- Nursing assistants need to follow the appropriate procedure if a patient falls.

NURSING ASSISTANT ALERT

Action	Benefit
Apply assistive devices carefully and correctly.	Contributes to patient's stability.
Use proper body mechanics when assisting a patient.	Avoids injury to patient and nursing assistant.
Learn the proper technique of two- and three-point gaits.	Provides knowledgeable support to patients who use canes and walkers.
Ensure that the wheelchair fits the patient.	Reduces the need for restraints, promotes independence in wheelchair mobility, and improves posture and body function.
Know and practice proper care and use of wheelchairs and stretchers.	Avoids accidents and injury to patients.

ACTIVITIES

Vocabulary Exercise

Write the words that form the circle on the left and their definitions on the right.

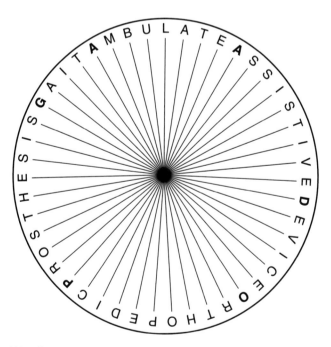

Word

1. _____

2. _____

3. _____

4. _____

5. _____

Definition

_____

_____

_____

_____

_____

Completion

Complete the following statements in the spaces provided. Select terms from the list provided.

affected	ambulation	arms	ball	four	heel
joint	need	rails	right	shoes	spills
strong	swinging	unsafe	90		

1. Walking is also known as _____.

2. In normal walking, the _____ strikes the floor before the _____ of the foot.

3. During walking, the arms normally have a slight _____ movement.

4. To walk safely, the patient must have adequate _____ motion.

5. The type of assistive device selected depends on a particular patient's _____.

6. Patients should be encouraged to use hand _____ when walking in the hallway.

7. When walking with a patient, the nursing assistant should stand on the patient's _____ side.

8. The nursing assistant should always check floors for clutter or _____.

9. No assistive device should be used if it is _____.

10. When forearm crutches with platforms are used, the elbows are constantly at a _____-degree angle to the shoulder.

11. When patients ambulate, clothes should not hang down over the _____.

12. A patient needs strength in both _____ to use a walker safely.

13. When ambulating with a walker, the patient shifts weight to the _____ leg as the walker is lifted and moved forward.

14. A wheelchair that fits properly will have about _____ inches between the top of the back and the patient's axillae.

15. When the feet are on the footrests of a wheelchair, the feet should be at a _____-degree angle to the legs.

True/False

Mark the following true or false by circling T or F.

1.   T   F   Before initiating an ambulation program, a physical therapist evaluates the patient.

2.   T   F   If a patient needs assistance but is using a cane, a gait belt need not be used.

3.   T   F   Quad canes provide a narrow base of support.

4.   T   F   Canes are recommended for aiding balance rather than providing support.

5.   T   F   A walker should be narrow so the patient can walk behind it.

6.   T   F   The walker can safely be used as a transfer device.

7.   T   F   Patients who are ambulating with a walker may use a two-point or three-point gait.

8.   T   F   A wheelchair that fits the patient properly will have a two- to three-inch clearance between the front edge of the seat and the back of the patient's knees.

9.   T   F   Pressure relief is not a concern for patients sitting in a chair or wheelchair.

10. T   F   A wheelchair is a transportation device.

Short Answer

Briefly answer the statements in the spaces provided.

1. Name three assistive devices that are commonly used for ambulation.

   a. _____

   b. _____

   c. _____

2. Explain why standard crutches are seldom recommended for older adults.

   _____

   _____

3. Explain the value of encouraging patients to do wheelchair push-ups.

   _____

   _____

4. List six guidelines for safely transporting a patient on a stretcher.

   a. _____

   b. _____

   c. _____

   d. _____

   e. _____

   f. _____

Clinical Situations

Briefly describe how a nursing assistant should react to the following situations.

1. Mrs. Keane is post-stroke and weak on her left side. She uses a walker when walking. You note that the hand grip is cracked and one of the bolt nuts is missing.

   _____

   _____

2. Mr. Jacks is using a walker for stability because he is still weak following abdominal surgery for colon cancer. You notice that he seems fatigued after walking the length of the corridor away from his room.

   _____

   _____

3. Mrs. De Koniger is ambulating with her walker. As she moves across the room, she moves her walker 15 inches in front of her, putting her weight on her weak leg as she brings her strong foot forward.

   _____

   _____

Identification

1. Circle the letter of the accompanying figure that shows the proper way to approach a closed door with a wheelchair.

A.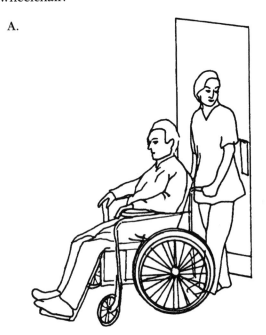

B.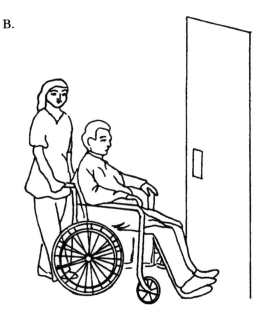

RELATING TO THE NURSING PROCESS

Write the step of the nursing process that is related to the nursing assistant action.

Nursing Assistant Action	Nursing Process Step
1. Two nursing assistants use a small sheet under the patient's buttocks to move the patient up in his wheelchair.	_____
2. The nursing assistant reports to the nurse that the patient wishes to ambulate but has only poorly fitting slippers at the bedside.	_____
3. The nursing assistant uses alcohol and cotton swabs to clean debris out of the ridges of a cane tip.	_____
4. The nursing assistant picks up old newspapers from the floor and disposes of them.	_____
5. The nursing assistant asks another assistant to make time to help ambulate Mr. Barker at 1:00 pm.	_____
6. The nursing assistant helps the therapist with the evaluation for gait training.	_____

DEVELOPING GREATER INSIGHT

Answer the following questions based on this situation.

Mrs. Stover is a 32-year-old patient whose tibia was fractured in an auto accident. The care plan states to ambulate her three times a day with the walker in the hallway, but the patient is depressed and often refuses. Several new approaches to motivate the patient are listed, and you try them. One of the new approaches is effective. Over the course of three days, Mrs. Stover improves her ambulation skills. She walked 15 feet with the walker on Tuesday. By Thursday, she is ambulating 50 feet with the walker, and minimum assistance with the gait belt. You inform the nurse of the effectiveness of the new approach and the patient's progress. During the next ambulation session, the nurse observes the patient and asks you to assist her with this evaluation. As a result of this assessment, the nurse holds a care plan conference to modify the plan of care. She invites you to attend to discuss the patient's progress and describe the patient's response to the approaches you used. You have noticed that the patient is likely to refuse ambulation during certain television programs, and suggest that the activity be scheduled to enable her to watch the shows she enjoys. List the actions used in caring for Mrs. Stover on the lines for the corresponding components of the nursing process.

1. Assessment

_____

_____

2. Planning

_____

_____

3. Implementation

_____

_____

4. Evaluation

_____

_____

Measuring and Recording Vital Signs, Height, and Weight

Body Temperature

OBJECTIVES

After completing this unit, you will be able to:

- Spell and define terms.
- Name and identify the types of clinical thermometers and describe their uses.
- Read a thermometer.
- Identify the range of normal temperature values.
- Demonstrate Procedures 25–29 (set out in this unit in the textbook).

UNIT SUMMARY

Temperature is the measurement of body heat. It varies in different areas in the same person.

- Average oral temperature is 98.6°F.
- Average rectal temperature is 99.6°F.
- Average axillary temperature is 97.6°F.

Temperature is measured in five areas of the body:

- Mouth (most common method)
- Underarm or groin (least accurate method)
- Rectum (most accurate *internal* method)
- Ear (high margin of error related to user technique)
- Forehead (rapid, accurate method with a wider range than other types of thermometers)

Measurements of temperature may be made using the Fahrenheit (F) or Celsius (centigrade or C) scale.

There are different-colored thermometer tips for rectal and oral use.

In addition to glass thermometers, there are other types of thermometers:

- The battery-operated electronic thermometer has different-colored tips for rectal and oral use.

- A plastic disposable oral thermometer has dots that change color according to the body temperature.

- With a tympanic thermometer, a probe placed in the external auditory canal measures body temperature at the tympanic membrane.

- With a digital thermometer, a probe is placed into the patient's mouth or rectum. This type of thermometer is battery-operated and the reading is shown as a digital display.

- With a temporal artery thermometer, the probe of the thermometer is scanned across the forehead and behind the ear. The reading is shown as a digital display.

The procedure for measuring body temperature should be carefully followed, including initial procedure actions and ending procedure actions.

NURSING ASSISTANT ALERT

Action	Benefit
Identify temperature values expressed in Fahrenheit scale.	Avoids error in measuring and recording temperature.
Be familiar with norms of temperature in different parts of the body.	Proper nursing actions can be taken when abnormal values are identified.
Use correct technique and procedures when taking temperatures.	Ensures accurate temperature values.
Cover glass thermometers and thermometer probes with disposable probe covers. Discard probe covers after single use.	Reduces the risk of spreading infection.
Hold glass and rectal, digital, tympanic, and axillary thermometers and probes in place.	Ensures accurate temperature measurement and avoids patient injury.
Be sure thermometers or probes are intact before insertion.	Prevents injury to the patient.
Record and report results accurately.	Ensures proper communication and evaluation of patient condition.

ACTIVITIES

Vocabulary Exercise

Define the words in the spaces provided.

1. temperature

_____

2. probe

_____

3. tympanic

_____

4. vital signs

_____

5. flagged

_____

Completion

Complete the statements in the spaces provided.

1. Measurement of body heat is one of the vital signs. Name three others.

    a. _____

    b. _____

    c. _____

2. When using an electronic thermometer, which part is inserted into the patient?

    _____

3. How is the part named in the previous question protected?

    _____

4. What happens to the protector after use?

    _____

5. Glass thermometers are long cylindrical tubes that contain a column of _____.

6. Each long line on a calibrated oral thermometer indicates an elevation of temperature of

    _____.

7. Each short line on the same thermometer indicates a rise in temperature of _____.

8. Three principles to keep in mind when reading a glass clinical thermometer are:

    a. _____

    b. _____

    c. _____

9. If the liquid column ends between two lines, it should be read to the _____.

10. Write the names of the two scales used to measure temperature.

    a. _____

    b. _____

11. What action should you take if the patient has just been smoking, drinking, or eating?

    _____

12. Before inserting a clean thermometer into the patient's mouth, you should

    a. _____

    b. _____

    c. _____

13. List three advantages of the tympanic thermometer.

    a. _____

    b. _____

    c. _____

14. Indicate which method of temperature determination (oral or rectal) is best in each of the following circumstances if only glass thermometers are available.

Method

a. Patient has diarrhea _____

b. Patient is confused _____

c. Patient cannot breathe through his nose _____

d. Patient has rectal bleeding _____

e. Patient is comatose _____

f. Patient has hemorrhoids _____

g. Patient is restless _____

h. Patient is a child _____

i. Patient has fecal impaction _____

j. Patient is coughing _____

15. Name two areas other than the mouth and rectum that can be used to determine body temperature.

a. _____

b. _____

16. Thermometers must be left in place for the proper amount of time to ensure recording. Write the time needed with each technique.

a. oral (glass thermometer) _____

b. rectal (glass thermometer) _____

c. axillary (glass thermometer) _____

d. tympanic thermometer _____

e. digital thermometer _____

f. temporal artery thermometer _____

17. Read the temperature measurement of each of the following glass thermometers.

Temperature Reading and Scale

a. _____

b. _____

c. _____

d. _____

e. _____

f. _____

g. _____

h. _____

i. _____

j. _____

18. Write the names of the thermometers pictured.

a. _____

b. _____

c. _____

d. _____

True/False

Mark the following true or false by circling T or F.

1. T F Body heat is managed by special cells in the liver.

2. T F The bulb of a rectal thermometer should always be lubricated before insertion.

3. T F Used glass thermometers should always be washed in hot soapy water before disinfection.

4. T F With an electronic thermometer, a new disposable probe cover should be used for each patient.

5. T F The probe of the tympanic thermometer should be placed directly under the patient's tongue.

6. T F A patient's temperature should be recorded as soon as it is taken.

Clinical Situations

1. Mrs. Morgan's oral temp was 98.4°F at 9:00 AM. When you see her at 10:30 AM, she is flushed and her skin is dry. What action should you take?

   _____

   _____

2. You are assigned to take the temperatures of two patients using the electronic thermometer. The sheath package is empty. You have only two temperatures to take and new sheaths are at the far end of the hall. What do you do?

   _____

   _____

RELATING TO THE NURSING PROCESS

Write the step of the nursing process that is related to the nursing assistant action.

Nursing Assistant Action	Nursing Process Step
1. The nursing assistant checks the glass thermometer carefully before placing it under the patient's tongue.	_____
2. The nursing assistant accurately reports that the patient's temperature is 102°F orally.	_____
3. Before inserting a glass clinical thermometer, the nursing assistant makes sure the liquid reads below 96°F.	_____
4. The nursing assistant checks the nursing care plan before measuring an oral temperature when she notices that the patient is receiving oxygen by face mask.	_____
5. The nursing assistant reports that the patient feels faint and has hot, flushed skin.	_____
6. The nursing assistant adjusts her assignment so she can recheck temperatures on patients with abnormal vital signs.	_____

DEVELOPING GREATER INSIGHT

Assume that you are caring for adult patients. Identify the values that should be reported to the nurse immediately with an R. Identify those that need not be reported immediately with an N.

1. 100.2°F (R) _____

2. 99.6°F (TAT) _____

3. 97.8°F (O) _____

4. 101.8°F (Ax) _____

5. 98.2°F (Ax) _____

6. 99.4°F (O) _____

7. 101.8°F (R) _____

8. 100.8°F (TAT) _____

Pulse and Respiration

OBJECTIVES

After completing this unit, you will be able to:

- Spell and define terms.
- Define pulse.
- Explain the importance of monitoring a pulse rate.
- Locate the pulse sites.
- Identify the range of normal pulse and respiratory rates.
- Measure the pulse at different locations.
- List the characteristics of the pulse and respiration.
- List eight guidelines for using the stethoscope.
- Demonstrate the procedures in the text.

UNIT SUMMARY

- Pulse and respiration rates and character are part of the vital signs.
- The pulse and respiration values are usually determined in a single procedure.
- Differences in apical and radial pulse rates are known as pulse deficits.

- Accurate values for respirations are best obtained when the patient is unaware that the procedure is being carried out.
- Unusual findings should be reported to the nurse.

NURSING ASSISTANT ALERT

Action	Benefit
Measure and record the character of pulse and respiration.	Provides important information regarding patient condition.
Recognize factors that alter pulse or respiratory rate.	Factors may be taken into account when evaluating findings.
Identify the norms for pulse and respiratory rates.	Proper nursing assistant actions may be taken when abnormal findings are identified.
Record findings accurately.	Ensures proper communication and evaluation of patient condition to other health care providers.

ACTIVITIES

Vocabulary Exercise

Each line has four different spellings of a word. Circle the correctly spelled word.

1. appical   apical   apecal   apicale
2. cyanosis   sianosis   syanosis   cyanoses
3. poulse   pullse   polse   pulse
4. despnea   dypnea   disnea   dyspnea
5. apnea   epnea   apnia   appnea
6. tachipnea   tachypnea   takipnea   tachipnia
7. rhythm   rhythem   rhethem   rytham
8. bradekardia   bradicardea   bradycardia   bradykardya

Completion

Complete the following statements in the spaces provided.

1. The pulse is the _____ of blood felt against the wall of an _____.

2. The pulse can be felt best in _____ that come close to the _____ and can be gently pressed against a _____.

3. When the patient is unconscious, you should measure the _____ or _____ pulse.

4. Pulse measurement includes determining the pulse character, which means the _____ and _____.

5. To check circulation to the toes of your patient with diabetes, you should palpate the _____ artery.

6. Seven major arteries used to measure pulse rates are:

a. _____

b. _____

c. _____

d. _____

e. _____

f. _____

g. _____

7. In an adult, the normal pulse rate is between _____ bpm and _____ bpm.

8. Your patient is 8 years old and has a pulse rate of 120. You know that this is _____ for a child of this age.

9. To accurately measure a pulse rate, your watch must have a _____.

10. You should locate the pulse with your _____.

11. The pulse should be counted for _____.

True/False

Mark the following true or false by circling T or F.

1. T   F   Normally the apical pulse is 4 bpm higher than the radial pulse in the same person.

2. T   F   Three health care providers are needed to accurately measure an apical pulse.

3. T   F   When determining an apical pulse, you will need a stethoscope.

4. T   F   The earpieces of the stethoscope must be cleaned before use.

5. T   F   Moist respirations are best documented as stertorous.

6. T   F   Each respiration consists of one inspiration and one expiration.

7. T   F   *Symmetry* of respirations refers to the depth of respiration.

8. T   F   The regularity of respirations is referred to as the *rhythm*.

9. T   F   The normal adult rate is 25 respirations per minute.

10. T   F   Always count the respiratory rate after you tell the patient what you intend to do.

Clinical Situations

Briefly describe how a nursing assistant should react to the following situations.

1. You are measuring vital signs and notice that the patient in 112B, whose pulse rate has been 84 to 88 bpm, now has a pulse rate of 112 and the pulse is weak.

_____

2. Mr. Murray has a medical diagnosis of congestive heart failure. When you measure his pulse, you find it irregular and weak. The nurse says she suspects a pulse deficit.

_____

3. You report that Mr. Rossi has a pulse deficit of 24 and a pulse rate of 84. What was the patient's apical pulse, and how would you document the reading? Show your work.

_____

4. Find the pulse deficit in each of the following readings and show proper documentation.

   a. apical pulse 120, radial pulse 104 _____

   b. apical pulse 118, radial pulse 88 _____

   c. apical pulse 92, radial pulse 50 _____

   d. apical pulse 102, radial pulse 68 _____

   e. apical pulse 98, radial pulse 76 _____

RELATING TO THE NURSING PROCESS

Write the step of the nursing process that is related to the nursing assistant action.

Nursing Assistant Action	Nursing Process Step
1. The nursing assistant tells the nurse that the patient's respirations have become more labored.	_____
2. The nursing assistant has an order to determine the apical pulse. She seeks help because she is not sure how to perform this procedure.	_____
3. The patient's pulse rate is 60 and the nursing assistant reports this information to the nurse.	_____
4. The nursing assistant listens closely as the nurse explains the new, revised care plans for the patients.	_____
5. The nursing assistant listens and counts the respirations for a full minute when the patient's respirations are irregular.	_____
6. The nursing assistant follows his assignment and obtains repeat vital signs for patients whose readings were abnormal 4 hours ago.	_____

DEVELOPING GREATER INSIGHT

Assume that you are caring for adult patients. Identify the values that should be reported to the nurse immediately with an R. Identify those that need not be reported immediately with an N.

1. P. 110, R. 24 _____

2. P. 96, R. 18 _____

3. P. 74, R. 20 _____

4. P. 52, R. 16 _____

5. P. 60, R. 28 _____

6. P. 68, R. 14 _____

7. P. 104, R. 20 _____

8. P. 88, R. 16 _____

Blood Pressure

OBJECTIVES

After completing this unit, you will be able to:

- Spell and define terms.
- Identify the range of normal blood pressure values.
- Identify the causes of inaccurate blood pressure readings.
- Select the proper size blood pressure cuff.
- List precautions associated with use of the sphygmomanometer.
- Describe the use of a pulse oximeter.
- Demonstrate Procedures 33 and 34 (set out in this unit in the textbook).

UNIT SUMMARY

Blood pressure must be determined and recorded accurately by watching the gauge of the sphygmomanometer and listening with the stethoscope.

- Note and record the first regular sound as the systolic pressure. This number represents the working pressure of the heart.

- Note and record the change in sound or the last sound as the diastolic pressure, as directed by facility policy. This number represents the resting pressure of the heart.

- Report unusual blood pressure to the nurse.

- Document the blood pressure as an improper fraction with the systolic reading above the diastolic reading.

Your bandage scissors, stethoscope, and other personal items may transfer pathogens from one patient to the next. If personal equipment items will be used during a procedure, wash them with an alcohol product or soap and water before and after each use. If you use a cloth stethoscope tubing cover, wash it each day with your uniform. Carry extra covers so you can change the cover if it becomes contaminated.

NURSING ASSISTANT ALERT

Action	Benefit
Use a blood pressure cuff of proper size.	Correct readings can be obtained only if the proper size cuff is used.
Clean stethoscope earpieces before and after use.	Prevents transmission of infection between caregivers.
Do not take blood pressure on an arm that has an IV or is paralyzed.	Prevents injury to the patient.
Read gauge at eye level.	Gives accurate reading.

ACTIVITIES

Vocabulary Exercise

Complete the puzzle by filling in the missing letters of words found in this unit. Use the definitions to help you discover these words.

```
                              H
1.                       _ Y _ _ _ _ _ _ _ _ _          1. low blood pressure

2.                       _ _ P _ _ _ _ _ _ _ _          2. high blood pressure

3.              _ _ _ _ _ _ E                           3. contraction of ventricles

4.                       _ R _ _ _ _ _ _                4. artery most often used to determine
                                                           blood pressure

5.                  _ _ _ _ T _ _ _ _ _                 5. stretchability

6.                       _ _ E _ _ _ _ _                6. type of gauge

7.  _ _ _ _ _ _ _ _ _ _ N _ _ _ _ _ _                  7. blood pressure cuff and gauge

8.                  _ _ S _ _ _ _ _ _ _ _ _ GAP        8. sound fadeout for 10 to 15 mm Hg,
                                                           after which sound begins again

9.          _ _ _ _ _ _ _ I _                           9. lowest blood pressure reading

10.     _ _ _ _ _ _ _ _ O _ _                          10. an instrument used to hear body
                                                           sounds
                              N
```

Completion

Write the answers in the spaces provided.

1. Blood pressure depends on four factors. List those factors.

    a. _____

    b. _____

    c. _____

    d. _____

2. When selecting a blood pressure cuff, make sure the bladder inside the cuff measures approximately _____ of the patient's arm.

3. Three types of sphygmomanometers in common use are:

   a. _____

   b. _____

   c. _____

4. The patient has a blood pressure reading of 148/98. You recognize this as _____.

5. The difference between the systolic and diastolic pressure is called the _____.

6. You should not use an arm to measure blood pressure if the arm is _____, the arm is the site of an _____, or the arm is _____.

7. Sound that fades out for 10 to 15 mm Hg and then resumes as you deflate the cuff is known as

   _____.

8. The large lines on the blood pressure gauge are at increments of _____ Hg.

9. Each small line on the blood pressure gauge indicates _____ intervals.

10. The cuff should be applied _____ above the elbow.

11. The center of the rubber bladder should be placed directly over the _____.

12. Three situations that you should immediately report regarding blood pressure measurement are:

   a. _____

   b. _____

   c. _____

13. Unusual blood pressure readings ought to be checked after _____.

14. Identify the equipment and the specific parts.

   a. _____

   b. _____

   c. _____

   d. _____

   e. _____

   f. _____

   g. _____

   h. _____

15. Determine the systolic and diastolic readings.

Systolic

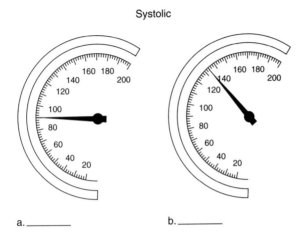

a. _____   b. _____

Diastolic

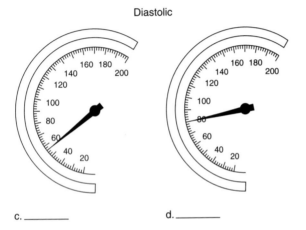

c. _____   d. _____

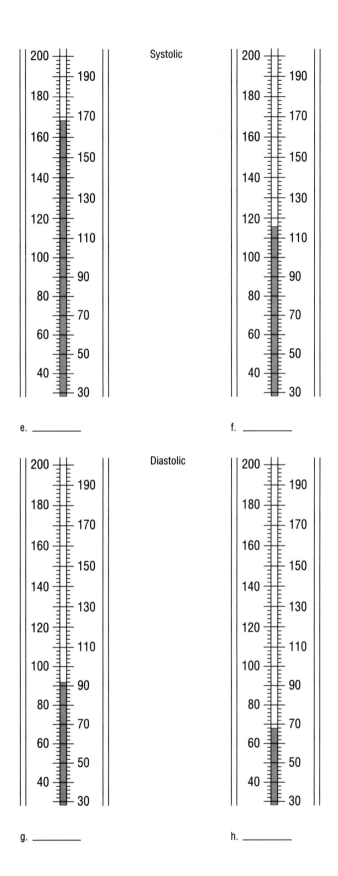

Systolic

e. _____

f. _____

Diastolic

g. _____

h. _____

True/False

Mark the following true or false by circling T or F.

1. T   F   The same size blood pressure cuff may be used for all patients.

2. T   F   The highest point of blood pressure measurement is the diastolic reading.

3. T   F   Deflating the cuff too slowly can result in an inaccurate reading.

4. T   F   All blood pressure readings should be made with the gauge above eye level.

5. T   F   The diastolic pressure is measured at the change sound or last sound that is heard.

6. T   F   The blood pressure is most often taken over the brachial artery.

7. T   F   Always clean the stethoscope earpieces and diaphragm before and after use.

8. T   F   Blood pressure readings are always recorded as a proper fraction such as 40/110.

9. T   F   It is very important to use a cuff of the correct size when determining the blood pressure.

10. T   F   A blood pressure measurement may be taken using an arm where an IV is inserted.

RELATING TO THE NURSING PROCESS

Write the step of the nursing process that is related to the nursing assistant action.

Nursing Assistant Action	Nursing Process Step
1. The nursing assistant finds that the patient's blood pressure is higher than the previous reading and reports this information.	_____
2. The patient is very heavy and the nursing assistant seeks guidance as to which size blood pressure cuff to use.	_____
3. The nursing assistant informs the team leader of the patient's vital signs before leaving for a break.	_____
4. The nursing assistant takes blood pressures as assigned.	_____

DEVELOPING GREATER INSIGHT

1. What action is taking place in the heart when you see the systolic reading?

_____

_____

2. Explain why narrowing of the blood vessels raises blood pressure.

_____

_____

3. Explain why a blood pressure cuff should not be placed on the same side as a recent mastectomy.

_____

_____

Measuring Height and Weight

OBJECTIVES

After completing this unit, you will be able to:

- Spell and define terms.
- List six nursing assistant actions to ensure that height and weight measurements are accurate.
- Identify at least four types of scales and give an example of when each type is used.
- Describe the proper use of an overbed scale.
- Demonstrate Procedure 35 (set out in this unit in the textbook).

UNIT SUMMARY

The patient's height and weight are usually measured at admission.

- Medications are often given according to the patient's weight.
- Weight changes may reflect the patient's condition and progress.

Measurements of height are made in:

- Feet (′)
- Inches (″)
- Centimeters (cm)

Measurements of weight are made in:

- Pounds (lb)
- Kilograms (kg)

Different techniques and equipment are used to make height and weight determinations, depending on the patient's condition.

NURSING ASSISTANT ALERT

Action	Benefit
Recognize that weight may be recorded in pounds or kilograms.	Prevents errors in measuring and documenting weights.
Remember that height can be measured in feet and inches or in centimeters.	Ensures correct interpretation of findings.
Always balance the scale before using.	Ensures that weight measurement is accurate.

ACTIVITIES

Vocabulary Exercise

The **boldfaced** and *italicized* words in the case study are hidden in the puzzle. Find them.

h	s	d	e	t	a	r	b	i	l	a	c
H	e	r	b	a	l	a	n	c	e	J	c
T	w	i	e	W	x	y	j	y	a	o	n
e	e	J	g	t	U	O	V	E	n	C	W
n	i	u	r	h	e	n	N	v	W	X	X
i	g	G	W	D	t	m	e	H	I	X	d
l	h	V	B	M	x	r	i	d	a	r	W
e	t	c	z	e	s	i	h	t	X	m	L
s	p	u	d	i	b	i	e	W	n	f	V
a	G	r	o	b	C	c	x	m	W	e	h
b	a	n	m	e	t	r	i	c	f	A	c
K	s	W	s	m	a	r	g	o	l	i	k

The nurse asks you to obtain a ***baseline height*** and ***weight*** on Mrs. Maciejewski, who was just admitted to your unit. You know that this means you are obtaining the initial values. Your facility uses metric values, so you will obtain the height in ***centimeters*** and the weight in ***kilograms***. No weight ***conversions*** are necessary, because the scales are ***calibrated*** for ***metric*** values. Before beginning the procedure, you remember to ***balance*** the scale so the weights hang free, to ensure that the value is accurate. When you have finished, you report to the nurse, who writes your findings on the ***Kardex***.

Completion

Complete the statements in the spaces provided. Select terms from the list provided.

bed	Chair	clothing	empty	kilograms
metric	paper towel	same	scale	
sling	tape measure	upright	wheelchair	

1. Choose the correct scale for each patient.

   a. Mr. Graham is in a wheelchair and cannot stand. He should be weighed with a/an _____ scale.

   b. Mrs. Almos is recovering from pneumonia and is up and about as desired. She should be weighed with a/an _____ scale.

   c. Mrs. DerHagopian is elderly. Her condition requires constant bedrest. She should be weighed with a/an _____ scale.

2. Patients should be weighed at the _____ time each day.

3. Patients should wear the same type of _____ each time they are weighed.

4. The same method and _____ should be used each time a patient is weighed.

5. Patients should _____ their bladders before being weighed.

6. When a patient cannot get out of bed, height measurement may be made with a _____.

7. Before you weigh a patient, cover the platform of an upright scale with a _____.

8. Some facilities use the _____ system, which records weights in _____.

Reading Weights and Heights

Read each weight measurement and record it in pounds.

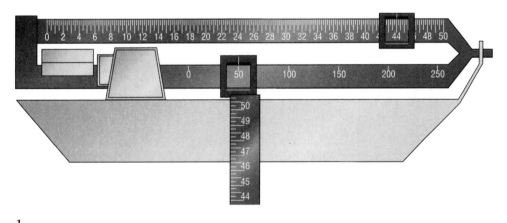

1. _____

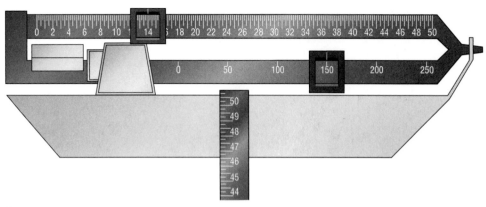

2. _____

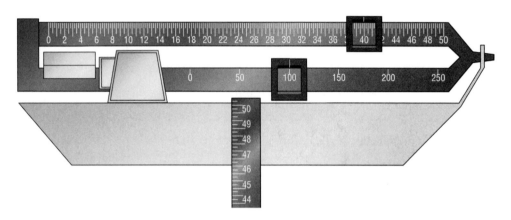

3. _____

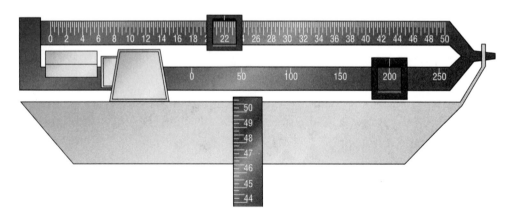

4. _____

Read each height measurement and record it in feet and inches.

5. _____

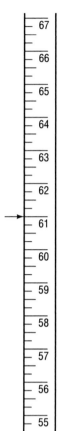

6. _____

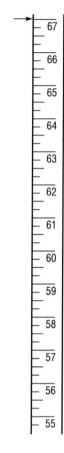

7. _____

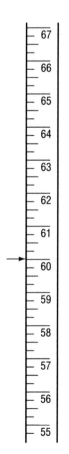

8. _____

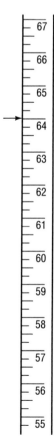

True/False

Mark the following true or false by circling T or F.

1.   T   F   Weights should be moved to the extreme left before weighing.

2.   T   F   Patients may hold the bar while being weighed as long as they do not lean on the scale.

3.   T   F   Before weighing a patient on a wheelchair scale, be sure to weigh the wheelchair only.

4.   T   F   The wheels of the wheelchair need not be locked when a patient is being weighed on a wheelchair scale.

5.   T   F   When a bed scale is used, the patient's body must be completely free of the bed before a reading is taken.

RELATING TO THE NURSING PROCESS

Write the step of the nursing process that is related to the nursing assistant action.

Nursing Assistant Action	Nursing Process Step
1. The nursing assistant measures and weighs Mrs. Maciejewski, a new patient, as instructed.	_____
2. To ensure that the weight measurement is accurate, the nursing assistant asks Mrs. Maciejewski to empty her bladder prior to weighing, to ensure that the weight is accurate.	_____
3. The nursing assistant assists Mrs. Maciejewski with toileting.	_____
4. The nursing assistant does not discard the urine. She asks the nurse if an admission urine specimen is needed. The nurse thanks her for thinking of this and asks her to take the specimen to the laboratory when she has finished with the height and weight procedures.	_____
5. After she has finished weighing Mrs. Maciejewski, the nursing assistant asists the patient to bed and helps make her comfortable.	_____
6. The nursing assistant reports Mrs. Maciejewski's height and weight to the nurse and records the measurements on the patient's record. The nurse records the height and weight on the Kardex.	_____
7. After Mrs. Maciejewski is comfortable and secure, the nursing assistant takes the urine specimen to the laboratory.	_____
8. The nurse starts an IV and administers an IV medication to eliminate fluid from the patient's legs. The following day, she asks the nursing assistant to weigh the patient again, compare the new measurement with the weight on the Kardex, and inform her if Mrs. Maciejewski has lost weight. If so, she would like to know the total amount of weight loss.	_____

DEVELOPING GREATER INSIGHT

Mrs. Arquilla is contracted in a fetal position. Her extremities are very tightly contracted and difficult to extend. You must obtain her height and weight.

1. How will you obtain an accurate height measurement for this patient?

_____

_____

_____

_____

2. You plan to use the electronic bed scale to weigh this patient. You place the sling and start to raise it off the surface of the bed when Mrs. Arquilla asks you to stop. She says, "I am too afraid. I might fall." What will you say to reassure her?

_____

_____

_____

_____

3. You persuade Mrs. Arquilla to let you finish the procedure, but she continues to yell when you raise the lift. Each time you stop and reassure her. What must you do to ensure that the weight measurement is accurate?

_____

_____

_____

_____

Patient Care and Comfort Measures

UNIT **22**

Admission, Transfer, and Discharge

OBJECTIVES

After completing this unit, you will be able to:

- Spell and define terms.
- List the ways the nursing assistant can help in the processes of admission, transfer, and discharge.
- List ways in which the nursing assistant can develop positive relationships with a patient's family members.
- Demonstrate Procedures 36–38 (set out in this unit in the textbook).

UNIT SUMMARY

The nursing assistant has specific responsibilities related to the admission, transfer, and discharge of the patient. These responsibilities include:

- Providing emotional support to both patient and family.
- Assisting in the safe physical transport of the patient.

- Carrying out the specific procedures relating to admission, transfer, and discharge.
- Preparing and disassembling the patient unit before and after use.
- Reporting and documenting observations.

NURSING ASSISTANT ALERT

Action	Benefit
Consider needs of visitors as well as those of the new patient.	Contributes to patient and family feelings of welcome and security.
Make careful observations and document accurately.	Provides information essential to the formulation of an appropriate nursing care plan.

ACTIVITIES

Vocabulary Exercise

Write the words forming the circle and define them. Start at the arrow.

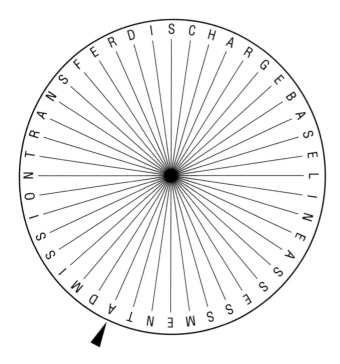

1. _____

_____

2. _____

_____

3. _____

_____

4. _____

_____

5. _____

_____

Completion

Complete the statements in the spaces provided.

1. Admission to a care facility is a cause of great concern for both _____ and
_____.

2. The nursing assistant should identify the patient by speaking her name and _____.

3. Jewelry and valuables not left at the cashier's office should be _____,
signed for, and sent home.

4. The nursing assistant can help orient the patient to the unit by explaining how to use the telephone
or television and the times _____ are served.

5. When transferring a patient to another unit, your manner should be _____ and
efficient.

6. Never leave the patient, his records, or his medications _____ during
the transfer procedure.

7. After a transfer is completed, you should be sure the patient is _____ and
_____.

8. Before preparing the patient for discharge, make sure the _____ has been written.

9. The nursing assistant's _____ are very valuable in the nurse's baseline assessment.

10. The patient is the facility's _____ until she has left the building.

11. After discharge, a final _____ is made on the patient chart.

12. Before the patient who is being discharged leaves, make sure the _____ have
been given to him.

Short Answer

Briefly answer the statements in the spaces provided.

1. The admission kit includes:

   a. _____

   b. _____

   c. _____

   d. _____

   e. _____

   f. _____

   g. _____

2. The nursing assistant can facilitate the admission procedure if seven points are kept in mind and carried
out. List them.

   a. _____

   b. _____

   c. _____

   d. _____

   e. _____

   f. _____

   g. _____

3. Before admitting the patient, you will need specific information. What questions should you ask the nurse?

a. _____

b. _____

c. _____

Clinical Situations

Briefly describe how a nursing assistant should react to the following situations.

1. Your patient tells you he intends to leave the health care facility without his physician's permission.

_____

2. Your patient has just been discharged.

_____

_____

_____

3. The family accompanies your patient to the unit and must wait as you carry out the admission procedure. How can you show courtesy to them?

_____

_____

_____

_____

_____

4. Your assignment is to admit the patient to Room 16C. Explain the equipment you will gather.

_____

_____

_____

_____

_____

RELATING TO THE NURSING PROCESS

Write the step of the nursing process that is related to the nursing assistant action.

Nursing Assistant Action	Nursing Process Step
1. The nursing assistant carefully prepares the patient's unit before admission.	_____
2. The nursing assistant measures the vital signs during the admission procedure.	_____
3. During admission, the nursing assistant carefully observes the patient and listens to the patient's statements.	_____
4. The nursing assistant makes sure that all the patient's personal articles are transported to the new unit when the patient is transferred.	_____
5. The nursing assistant documents the correct time and method of patient discharge on the proper record.	_____

DEVELOPING GREATER INSIGHT

You are assigned to admit a new 71-year-old dependent patient who has been cared for in the home of family members. Her daughter talks nonstop and gives you advice on caring for the patient. The patient cannot speak, but her facial expression and body language suggest that she is afraid. You notice that the patient has open areas on both hips. She has bruises on her arms. She is wearing an incontinent brief. The patient has dried stool on her bottom, and smells of urine. Her teeth are in poor repair and she has remnants of food in her mouth and on her clothing. The patient's tongue and oral mucous membranes appear very dry. The patient is 66 inches tall and weighs 87 pounds.

1. What does this patient's appearance suggest?

_____

_____

2. What action will you take?

_____

_____

Bedmaking

OBJECTIVES

After completing this unit, you will be able to:

- Spell and define terms.
- Operate each type of bed.
- Properly handle clean and soiled linens.
- Demonstrate Procedures 39–42 (set out in this unit in the textbook).

UNIT SUMMARY

Proper bedmaking is an important part of your work. A skillfully made bed provides comfort and safety for the patient.

Beds may be built to meet specific patient needs and conditions. Each type of bed will be made differently. Types of beds include:

- Electric
- Gatch
- Low
- Various specialty beds

Bedmaking methods include:

- Closed bed
- Occupied bed
- Unoccupied bed
- Surgical bed

Drawsheets or turning sheets may be used, depending on patient requirements. In some facilities, large reusable underpads are used in place of turning sheets.

Some facilities use fitted bottom sheets. The bedmaking procedure may be modified to accommodate this difference.

NURSING ASSISTANT ALERT

Action	Benefit
Handle linen carefully and properly.	Prevents spread of germs.
Raise bed to comfortable working height during procedure.	Reduces strain on caregiver.
Make bed neatly and smoothly.	Contributes to comfort and lessens chance of (pressure) ulcer formation.
Know how to operate bed and equipment before attempting to do so.	Avoids injury to patient and caregiver.
Always leave bed in lowest horizontal position.	Reduces the possibility of accidents when patient gets in and out of bed.
Use standard precautions if contact with blood, body fluids, secretions, or excretions is likely.	Prevents spread of germs. Protects caregiver.
Follow all safety precautions when making low beds.	Prevents caregiver strain and back injury.

ACTIVITIES

Vocabulary Exercise

Unscramble the words introduced in this unit and define them.

1. C U B R I L D E S G A _____

_____

2. H A C G T _____

_____

3. U R E S O C R E Q A N R _____

_____

4. I E T D R E M _____

_____

5. T E P A O L E T _____

_____

6. I R S E A D L I S _____

_____

7. E T H E S _____

_____

True/False

Mark the following true or false by circling T or F.

1.   T   F   After the bottom of the bed has been made, you then pull the mattress to the head of the bed.

2.   T   F   Before making a bed, lower it to its lowest horizontal height.

3.   T   F   When completing an open bed, the top bedding is positioned to the top of the bed under the pillow.

4. T F The top linen of a surgical bed is left untucked and fanfolded to one side.

5. T F A lift sheet should be positioned from the patient's waist to his knees.

6. T F The electrically operated bed is the type of bed most commonly found in an acute care facility.

7. T F A mattress pad is applied to the mattress before the bottom sheet.

8. T F Fitted sheets are used in some facilities in place of top sheets.

9. T F Before making an unoccupied bed, arrange the linen in the order it is to be used.

10. T F Always position a patient comfortably before leaving the room.

11. T F The flat bottom sheet should be placed so the bottom edge is even with the end of the mattress at the foot of the bed.

12. T F Linen to make a bed should be placed on the overbed table.

13. T F Never shake the linen when making a bed, because this may spread germs.

14. T F When making the bottom of an occupied bed, the linen should be rolled against the patient's back and then tucked under the patient's body.

15. T F The top linen should be loosened when a bed is occupied.

16. T F Side rails should be up and secure before you leave an occupied bed.

Identification

Identify the following items.

1. Name the type of corner that has been made in the linen.

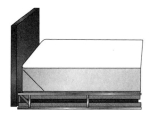

_____

2. Identify the type of bed pictured here.

_____

2   3

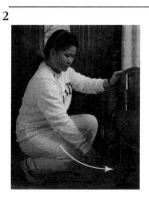
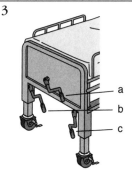

3. State the purpose of each handle at the foot of the bed.

   a. _____

   b. _____

   c. _____

4. Identify the items pictured here.

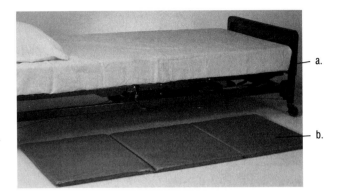

a. _____

b. _____

5. Name the fold the nursing assistant is making in the linen.

a. _____

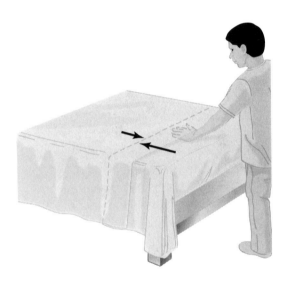

b. State the purpose of folding the linen in this manner.

_____

Short Answer

Briefly answer the following questions.

1. Why should one side of the bed be made at a time?

_____

2. Why are the sheets unfolded rather than shaken out?

_____

3. How should the pillow be placed on the bed?

_____

4. What is the purpose of the open bed?

_____

5. What is the purpose of the surgical bed?

_____

6. Why is it important to screen the patient unit before beginning to make an occupied bed?

_____

7. How will you learn whether the patient's side rails should be pulled up or left down when you leave the room?

_____

8. What is the proper position for the overbed table when the bed is closed or unoccupied?

_____

9. When is the closed bed made in the hospital?

_____

10. Why would the wheels of the bed be locked before you start to make the bed?

_____

Completion

Complete the following chart.

Method of Bedmaking	Procedure Variations	Rationale
Unoccupied Bed	1. Most _____ type of bedmaking procedure • Used for making all types of beds	2. Making the unoccupied bed is _____ and faster for the nursing assistant. It is more comfortable for the patient.
Occupied Bed	3. Used when the patient is _____ to bed.	Changes wet or soiled linen for patient comfort and prevention of skin breakdown. Provides fresh, clean linen for feeling of comfort and security.
4. _____ Bed	• The bed is made with the top sheet, blanket, and spread pulled all the way to the top. • The pillow may be covered or placed on top of the spread, depending on facility policy. • The open end of the pillowcase faces away from the door.	5. Used when the patient is expected to be _____ all day or when making a bed after a patient has been discharged. Presents a neat, tidy appearance.
Open Bed	• The bed is made in the normal manner. 6. The top sheet and spread are _____ to the foot of the bed.	This procedure is used when the patient is temporarily out of bed. The patient or nursing assistant can easily and quickly cover the patient upon return to bed.

Clinical Situations

Briefly describe how a nursing assistant should react to the following situations.

1. You finish making the occupied bed and you notice that the bed is at the working (elevated) horizontal height.

   _____

2. You took a clean towel into the patient's room and found that it was not needed. What should you do with the towel?

   _____

Answer the questions about the clinical situation. Briefly explain your answers.

It is career day for your local high school. The nurse manager of your unit has asked you to allow a high school student to "shadow" you during your shift. You know that only the best workers are asked to work with these students and you feel honored to be asked. The student, who is close to your age, is glad to be there and very excited to be working with you. She has many questions. The student asks you the following:

3. What is the purpose of the low bed in room 321?

   _____

   _____

4. What is the purpose of the mat on the floor next to the low bed?

   _____

   _____

5. Doesn't it hurt your back to care for the patient in the low bed and make the bed while bending over? What can you do to prevent a backache?

   _____

   _____

   _____

   _____

   _____

6. Why do you elevate the electric hospital bed when you are making the bed?

   _____

   _____

7. Why do you lower the bed when you have finished making it?

   _____

   _____

8. Why did you leave the room to put the soiled bed linen in the hamper in the hallway? Wouldn't it be easier to put it on the floor and take it to the hamper when you have finished?

   _____

   _____

   _____

9. What is the purpose of the half sheet in the center of the bed?

   _____

   _____

10. After you finished making the bed, you pulled the top linen down and folded it at the foot of the bed. That seems like undoing what you just finished. Why did you do this?

_____

_____

_____

_____

RELATING TO THE NURSING PROCESS

Write the step of the nursing process that is related to the nursing assistant action.

Nursing Assistant Action	Nursing Process Step
1. The nursing assistant makes sure the bottom bed linen is free of wrinkles.	_____
2. The nursing assistant accompanies the nurse so the assistant can help turn a patient on a special therapeutic bed.	_____
3. The nursing assistant makes sure the patient is not exposed when the bed linen is changed.	_____
4. The nursing assistant is assigned to prepare a bed for a postoperative patient. Because she has not done this before, she asks the nurse for clarification.	_____
5. The nursing assistant replaces the drawsheet with a large underpad to see if using the pad makes it easier to turn the patient.	_____
6. Mr. Neufeld is paralyzed on the left side of his body. He is right handed. There are 4 half rails on the bed. The two upper rails are elevated. The lower rails are not used. Mr. Neufeld has a care plan goal to learn to pull on the side rails to assist with bed mobility. The patient turns well from side to side, but cannot sit up in bed by pulling on the upper rails. The nursing assistant raises the right lower rail and shows the patient where to place his hand. He pulls himself up in bed.	_____
7. The nursing assistant informs the nurse of Mr. Neufeld's ability to sit up if the lower rail is raised. The nurse adds the information to the care plan.	_____
8. The nurse watches as the assistant works with Mr. Neufeld on bed mobility. She notes that the patient is pleased with his progress. The nurse thanks the nursing assistant for teaching him the new approach, which he uses successfully.	_____

DEVELOPING GREATER INSIGHT

Mr. Leveque is a dependent patient in a low bed. The care plan states he is a two-person transfer. One side of his bed is next to the wall. There is a large plastic mat on the floor on the open side of the bed.

1. What safety precautions will you take to prevent injury to patient and staff when assisting him into and out of bed?

_____

_____

_____

_____

Patient Bathing

OBJECTIVES

After completing this unit, you will be able to:

- Spell and define terms.
- Describe the safety precautions for patient bathing.
- List the purposes of bathing patients.
- Demonstrate Procedures 43–51 (set out in this unit in the textbook).

UNIT SUMMARY

Bathing makes a patient feel refreshed and clean. Full or partial baths may be carried out in:

- Bed
- Shower
- Regular bathtub
- Whirlpool tub

Personal hygiene measures include:

- Care of the teeth
- Care of the hair
- Care of the nails
- Dressing and undressing

Patients should be encouraged to participate in personal hygiene measures and the choice of garments. Range-of-motion exercises are frequently performed during the bath procedure, according to the patient's needs and orders. The daily hygiene routine gives you a chance to make close observations of the patient.

NURSING ASSISTANT ALERT

Action	Benefit
Guard against falls.	Avoids potential injury.
Maintain an even room temperature.	Prevents chilling and discomfort.
Avoid unnecessary exposure.	Protects patient's dignity and privacy.
Work quickly and smoothly, using proper body mechanics.	Lessens patient and caregiver fatigue.

ACTIVITIES

Vocabulary Exercise

Each line has four different spellings of a word. Circle the correctly spelled word.

1. cutical	cuticule	cuticale	cuticle
2. axillae	axiller	axella	arxilla
3. genetala	genitalia	genetalea	ginetalia
4. perineanum	pirineam	perineum	perinium
5. pubic	pubec	pobic	paobic

Completion

Complete the statements in the spaces provided.

1. A daily bath makes the patient feel _____ and clean.

2. In addition to bathing the body, morning care includes cleaning the teeth, _____, and _____.

3. A partial bath ensures cleansing of the hands, face, _____, buttocks, and _____.

4. The best temperature for bath water is about _____°F.

5. A _____ should be in the bath area in case of an emergency.

6. After the tub bath is completed and the patient has returned to the unit, return to the tub room and _____ the tub.

7. To provide privacy during a tub bath or shower, the patient may use a _____ to wrap around his _____.

8. As the patient steps out of the tub, hold a _____ around the patient to provide privacy.

9. During a bed bath, privacy can be provided by _____.

10. Before the bed bath, you should offer the patient a _____.

11. When preparing the patient for a bed bath, remove the top bedding and replace it with a _____.

12. Do not use soap near the _____.

13. When cleaning the eyes, always wipe from _____ to _____ corner.

14. Pay special attention to the folds under a female patient's _____ as you wash her.

15. A bag bath may be used instead of using _____.

16. Apply _____ to the feet of a patient with dry skin.

17. When clipping fingernails, clip the nails _____ and do not clip below the _____.

18. When finishing the bath for the male patient, carefully wash and dry the _____, _____, and groin area.

19. The whirlpool tub provides the beneficial action of a _____ in addition to cleaning.

20. When giving a bed shampoo, _____ the scalp with your _____.

21. During a bed shampoo, give the patient a _____ to protect the patient's eyes.

22. Dry the hair following a shampoo with a _____ or portable hair dryer.

Short Answer

Briefly answer the following questions.

1. Three values patients derive from a bath include:

   a. _____

   b. _____

   c. _____

2. Three precautions you should take when the patient is able to bathe himself in a tub include:

   a. _____

   b. _____

   c. _____

3. Special care must be given during the bath to the patient who:

   a. _____

   b. _____

   c. _____

4. Describe how you should remove the gown of a patient who is receiving an intravenous infusion in order to bathe the patient.

   a. _____

   b. _____

   c. _____

   d. _____

   e. _____

   f. _____

5. Describe how a bath mitt is made.

   _____

   _____

   _____

6. List three advantages to using the waterless bathing system compared with a regular bed bath.

   a. _____

   b. _____

   c. _____

7. Why should the patient help you with the bed bath as much as his condition permits?

   _____

   _____

8. What is the nursing assistant's responsibility when the patient is unable to complete the bath by herself?

   _____

   _____

9. What other procedures may be carried out in conjunction with the bath procedure?

_____

_____

10. What are four advantages of the whirlpool bath?

    a. _____

    b. _____

    c. _____

    d. _____

11. What measures can be taken to help avoid patient falls during tub bathing?

_____

_____

_____

Clinical Situations

Briefly describe how a nursing assistant should react to the following situations.

1. Your patient feels weak or faint during a tub bath.

_____

_____

2. You have not yet finished bathing the legs of a bed patient and the water feels cool.

_____

_____

3. Your patient has diabetes and his toenails need to be cut.

_____

_____

4. Describe the technique to be used when washing the penis and scrotum.

_____

_____

RELATING TO THE NURSING PROCESS

Write the step of the nursing process that is related to the nursing assistant action.

Nursing Assistant Action   **Nursing Process Step**

1. The nursing assistant carefully cleans the tub before and after each patient use.   _____

2. The nursing assistant has to bathe a patient with an IV line and is not sure how to remove the patient's gown. She asks a nurse for help.   _____

3. The nursing assistant offers a bedpan to the patient before giving a bed bath.   _____

4. The nursing assistant finds that the patient cannot separate her legs sufficiently to allow good perineal care, so the assistant asks the nurse for directions on how to give care.   _____

5. The nursing assistant is giving foot care to a patient with thick, long toenails. He asks the nurse if the nails should be cut.   _____

6. The nursing assistant listens carefully as the nurse explains that the care plan for a bed bath will be modified the next day to allow the patient to shower if she feels well enough.   _____

7. The nursing assistant carefully checks the patient's skin during the bathing procedure.   _____

General Comfort Measures

After completing this unit, you will be able to:

- Spell and define terms.
- Discuss the reasons for early morning and bedtime care.
- List the purposes of oral hygiene.
- Identify patients who require frequent oral hygiene.
- Explain nursing assistant responsibilities for a patient's dentures.
- State the purpose of backrubs.
- Describe safety precautions when shaving a patient.
- Describe the importance of hair care.
- Explain the use of comfort devices.
- Demonstrate Procedures 52–57 (set out in this unit in the textbook).

UNIT SUMMARY

You can take several measures to add to the patient's general comfort. These measures include:

- Caring for the patient's teeth and hair
- Shaving the patient
- Giving backrubs to soothe and stimulate
- Meeting elimination needs promptly and providing privacy

Early morning or AM care:

- Refreshes the patient before breakfast
- Prepares the patient for the day

Bedtime or PM care is a similar procedure that is followed in the evening before sleep. It helps the patient to relax and prepare for sleep.

NURSING ASSISTANT ALERT

Action	Benefit
Carry out hygiene measures that patients cannot do for themselves.	Improves patient comfort.
Encourage patients to assist when possible.	Builds self-esteem and supports independence.
Give AM care in a pleasant manner.	Sets a positive tone for the day.
Provide PM care in an unrushed manner.	Helps patients relax and be more inclined to sleep.
Provide privacy.	Contributes to patient's emotional security.
Meet elimination needs promptly.	Reduces patient discomfort. Aids in promoting normal elimination.

ACTIVITIES

Vocabulary Exercise

In the word puzzle, find each term defined in the following list. Circle the term in the puzzle.

h	u	s	e	c	e	f	s	c
x	a	d	a	c	o	e	p	a
h	t	l	j	k	r	b	d	r
l	h	q	i	u	j	c	t	i
j	k	s	t	t	o	p	z	e
y	a	n	y	y	o	r	u	s
p	e	i	b	w	l	s	a	u
d	j	x	h	w	o	u	i	l
l	b	u	r	k	c	a	b	s

1. false teeth

2. massage of the back

3. unpleasant breath

4. care of mouth and teeth is _____ hygiene

5. dental cavities

6. solid waste

Completion

Complete the following statements in the spaces provided.

1. When out of the mouth, dentures should be stored in a _____

   _____ .

2. Lubricant is applied to the lips for _____

   _____ .

3. Dentures should be handled _____ to prevent damage.

4. The denture storage container should be labeled with _____

   _____ .

5. Proper mouth cleaning helps prevent halitosis and dental _____ .

6. A toothbrush should be inserted into the mouth with the bristles in a _____ position.

7. Special oral hygiene is given by using _____ or _____ .

8. Lubricant is usually applied to the lips with _____ .

9. If possible, the patient should be in a(n) _____ position during toothbrushing.

10. To protect dentures during cleaning, always _____ .

11. Before giving a backrub, _____ lotion in _____ .

12. A special order may be needed to shave the face of a patient who is taking _____ .

13. When shaving a patient's face, the skin should be held _____ .

14. Brushing the hair makes the patient feel better and _____ the scalp.

15. Before breakfast, the patient should be given the opportunity to go to the bathroom or to use the

    _____ .

16. Evening care should be given in a _____ , _____ manner.

17. During evening care, be sure to clear the _____ table and adjust the
    _____ of the bed.

18. Part of AM and PM care includes tightening the _____ and straightening the
    _____ linen.

19. After PM care, the bed should be in the _____ horizontal position if the
    patient's condition permits.

Short Answer

Briefly answer the following questions.

1. Why is oral hygiene important?

   _____

2. Why are frequent backrubs important to the patient who is not permitted out of bed?

   _____

3. Why should nursing assistants keep their fingernails short?

   _____

4. Why should the skin be held taut while you are using a razor?

   _____

5. What would you do if you accidentally nicked a patient during the shaving procedure?

_____

6. What action would you take if the patient's hair was tangled?

_____

7. Why must gloves be worn when shaving a patient's intact face with a disposable razor?

_____

8. Six patients requiring special oral hygiene are those who are:

 a. _____

 b. _____

 c. _____

 d. _____

 e. _____

 f. _____

9. List five times when backrubs are usually given.

 a. _____

 b. _____

 c. _____

 d. _____

 e. _____

10. List the equipment you would need to give a backrub.

 a. _____

 b. _____

 c. _____

 d. _____

11. Why is mouth care given before the patient has breakfast?

_____

12. Why is a backrub given to the patient at bedtime?

_____

13. How do you wake a patient?

_____

14. Name two instances when you would not waken the patient.

 a. _____

 b. _____

15. Identify four activities you will carry out as part of bedtime care.

 a. _____

 b. _____

 c. _____

 d. _____

Identifying Strokes

Using a colored pencil or crayon, draw in the indicated strokes.

1. Soothing

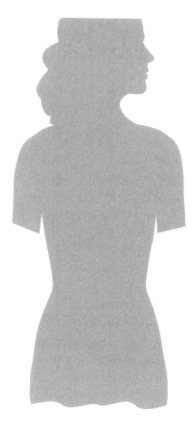

2. Passive

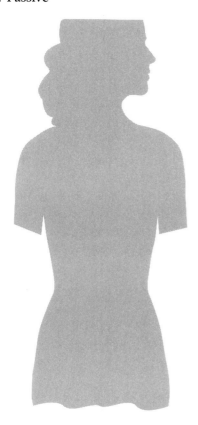

3. Circular

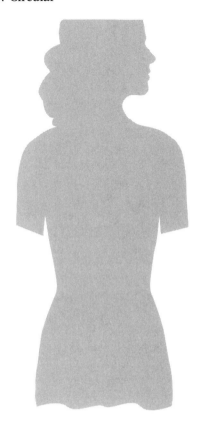

True/False

Mark the following true or false by circling T or F.

1. T F Never place a bedpan on the overbed table.

2. T F Place the bedpan cover on the bedside stand.

3. T F Warm the bedpan by filling it with very hot water.

4. T F You do not need to cover a used bedpan if the bathroom is close to the patient's room.

5. T F A small folded towel can be used to pad a bedpan if the patient is very thin.

6. T F If the patient is very heavy, you may need assistance placing him on a bedpan.

7. T F The patient's buttocks should rest on the narrow end of the fracture bedpan.

8. T F The curtains should be drawn around a patient who is using a bedpan.

9. T F Make sure the signal cord is close at hand when the patient is on a bedpan.

10. T F Bedpan contents should be noted and documented.

Name the Equipment

Enter the name of the equipment pictured in the space provided.

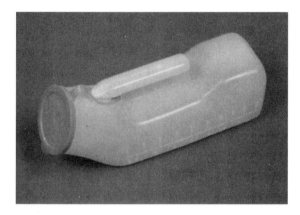

1. _____

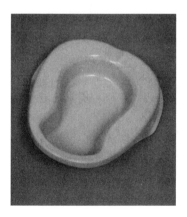

2. _____

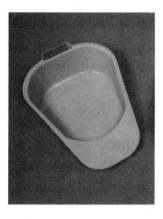

3. _____

Clinical Situations

Briefly describe how a nursing assistant should react to the following situations.

1. You note a pressure area on your patient's hip while giving a backrub.

   _____

   _____

2. You must do a bed shampoo to wash the hair of an African American patient who vomited while in bed. Some of the vomitus accidentally got into her hair. The patient has a comb, brush, and elastic hair ties, but did not bring any hair care products to the facility. What hair care products will you need to wash, detangle, dry, and style her hair?

   _____

   _____

   _____

3. Your patient needs to use the bedpan, but cannot lift her buttocks off the bed.

   _____

   _____

4. You are giving PM care and the patient says he would like to finish the chapter he is reading.

   _____

5. Your patient is scheduled for surgery at 9:00 AM and you are assigned to provide AM care to the patient in her room.

   _____

6. Your patient is settled for the night and you are ready to leave the room.

   _____

RELATING TO THE NURSING PROCESS

Write the step of the nursing process that is related to the nursing assistant action.

Nursing Assistant Action	Nursing Process Step
1. The nursing assistant allows the patient to sleep and omits early AM care because the patient is going to surgery.	_____
2. The nursing assistant makes sure that bedtime care has been given before the nurse administers sleep medications.	_____
3. The nursing assistant uses cool water when brushing the patient's dentures.	_____
4. The nursing assistant reports that the patient's lips are very dry and cracked.	_____
5. The nursing assistant listens carefully when the patient says that he does not want to put his dentures in because they hurt.	_____
6. The nursing assistant reports and documents the condition of the patient's skin each time she gives back care.	_____

Principles of Nutrition, Hydration, and Elimination

UNIT **26**

Urinary Elimination

OBJECTIVES

After completing this unit, you will be able to:

- Spell and define terms.
- Identify aging changes of the urinary system.
- List some common diseases of the urinary system.
- Identify signs and symptoms of the urinary system that the nursing assistant must observe and report.
- Describe nursing assistant actions related to the care of patients with urinary system diseases and conditions.
- Demonstrate Procedures 58–71 (set out in this unit in the textbook).

UNIT SUMMARY

Two nursing measures are vital in the care of patients with urinary dysfunction:

- Maintaining adequate urinary drainage
- Keeping drainage equipment free of contamination

The urinary tract is considered a sterile area. Special sterile techniques must be used when the physician or nurse introduces a catheter into this area. The nursing assistant must know how to safely:

- Disconnect the catheter from the drainage setup
- Empty and measure the drainage
- Ambulate the patient who has constant urinary drainage

NURSING ASSISTANT ALERT

Action	Benefit
Secure and care for urine specimens according to policy.	Contributes to more accurate data.
Maintain patency in the urinary drainage system.	Prevents backup of urine and subsequent damage.
Maintain accurate I&O records.	Helps to monitor renal function.
Protect drainage tubing connection sites.	Keeps drainage system free from contamination.
Keep drainage bag below level of bladder.	Prevents reflux of drained urine into the bladder.

ACTIVITIES

Vocabulary Exercise

Complete the crossword puzzle using the clues below.

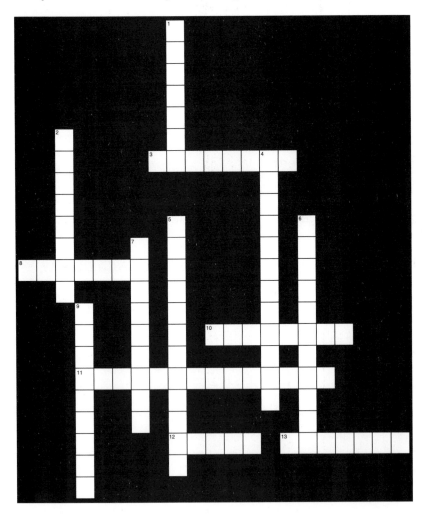

Across

3 Removal of waste products from the blood with an artificial kidney machine

8 Renal _____ is the inability of the kidneys to maintain fluid and electrolyte balance, excrete waste, and regulate essential body functions.

10 Inflammation of the bladder

11 A condition resulting from too much fluid on the kidney

12 Renal _____ causes severe renal pain.

13 Painful urination

Down

1 Kidney stones

2 Decreased urine production

4 Infection and _____ are the most common conditions of the urinary system.

5 Loss of control over urination; involuntary urination

6 Procedure that uses sound waves to crush kidney stones

7 Blood in the urine

9 Inflammation of one or both kidneys

Definitions

Define the terms or abbreviations.

1. dysuria

_____

2. hematuria

_____

3. hydronephrosis

_____

4. kidneys

_____

5. retention

_____

6. ureter

_____

7. nephritis

_____

8. cystitis

_____

Completion

Complete the following statements in the spaces provided.

1. Fluid intake should be _____ in patients with renal calculi.

2. The average adult requires at least _____ of fluid each day to maintain kidney function.

3. You might expect the blood pressure of a patient with long-standing renal disease to be _____.

4. Renal calculi can cause _____ to the normal flow of urine.

5. All the urine of a patient with renal calculi should be _____.

6. The patient with renal calculi should have fluids _____.

7. Lithotripsy is a technique used to _____ renal calculi.

8. The Foley catheter has a _____ surrounding the neck so the catheter can be retained in the bladder.

9. Insertion of a catheter is a _____ procedure and should be performed by the _____ or _____.

10. Urinary condoms can be used on _____ patients who need long-term drainage.

11. Avoid disconnecting the _____, if possible.

12. Special care is needed for patients who have urinary conditions, because the urinary tract is a _____ area.

13. If a sample of urine cannot be delivered to the laboratory immediately, it should be _____.

14. Approximately _____ of urine are sent to the laboratory as a specimen.

15. Before collecting a midstream urine specimen, always clean the area around the _____ and then allow some urine to be expelled.

16. The procedure for collection of a 24-hour urine specimen requires that the patient start the 24-hour interval with the bladder _____.

17. The last urine voided is _____ in the 24-hour specimen.

Short Answer

Briefly answer the following questions.

1. List four things the nursing assistant is expected to do in the care of a patient who is receiving dialysis treatments.

    a. _____

    b. _____

    c. _____

    d. _____

2. Most adults take in _____ of fluid daily.

3. When the patient does not consume sufficient fluid, kidney filtration is slow, causing waste products to be _____.

4. If you serve nourishments to a resident on I&O, you must _____.

5. What are two common types of catheters used to drain the urinary bladder?

    a. _____

    b. _____

6. What are seven responsibilities of nursing assistant who is caring for a patient with urinary drainage?

   a. _____

   b. _____

   c. _____

   d. _____

   e. _____

   f. _____

   g. _____

7. If urinary drainage must be disconnected, what parts must be protected against contamination?

   a. _____

   b. _____

Clinical Situations

Briefly describe how a nursing assistant should react to the following situations.

1. Your patient has an indwelling catheter. Explain the daily care you will provide.

   _____

   _____

   _____

2. Your patient uses condom drainage. List three responsibilities of the nursing assistant.

   a. _____

   b. _____

   c. _____

3. Your patient is on I&O. Explain how to measure the drainage when the patient has an indwelling catheter.

   _____

   _____

4. Your patient has urinary drainage into a leg bag. List four points to keep in mind while providing care.

   a. _____

   b. _____

   c. _____

   d. _____

5. _____ is a very serious condition in the elderly. Patients who are at high risk for this condition have not consumed enough liquid to support their minimum body functions.

6. One ounce of liquid is the approximate equivalent of _____ mL (cc).

7. One quart of liquid is the approximate equivalent of _____ mL (cc).

8. When recording I&O, count all fluids and food items that become _____ at room temperature.

RELATING TO THE NURSING PROCESS

Write the step of the nursing process that is related to the nursing assistant action.

Nursing Assistant Action	Nursing Process Step
1. The nursing assistant promptly reports that the patient is experiencing chills.	_____
2. The nursing assistant checks the drainage tubing to be sure that it is fastened properly and is not obstructed.	_____
3. The nursing assistant plans time to provide catheter care during the patient's bath.	_____
4. The nursing assistant wears gloves when handling the patient's urinary drainage equipment.	_____
5. The nursing assistant strains all urine as ordered when the patient has renal calculi.	_____
6. The nursing assistant saves a particle found in the paper urine filter and informs the nurse so the nurse can evaluate it.	_____
7. If the patient is not circumcised, the nursing assistant makes sure to reposition the foreskin after giving indwelling catheter care.	_____
8. The nursing assistant maintains a positive attitude when changing the soiled linen of a patient who is incontinent.	_____
9. All the nursing assistants add urine to a 24-hour collection from a single patient even though the patient is the primary responsibility of one nursing assistant.	_____
10. The nursing assistant totals the intake and output, documents it on the I&O record, and informs the nurse.	_____

DEVELOPING GREATER INSIGHT

Calculate the total fluid intake for each patient.

1. Mrs. Holiday drank 3 ounces water + 4 ounces coffee + 3 ounces juice + 240 mL milk.

_____

2. Mr. Gomez consumed 8 ounces fruit drink + 6 ounces soup + 5 ounces tea + ½ cup ice cream.

_____

3. Miss Stockburger consumed 300 mL water + 8 ounces supplement + 16 ounces soda + ½ cup gelatin.

_____

4. Mrs. Schoebel drank 4 ounces tea + 8 ounces milk + 1 ounce cream + 4 ounces juice.

_____

5. Mrs. Sedala consumed a 4-ounce cup of sherbet + 12 ounces milk + 6 ounces coffee.

_____

6. Mr. Frahler drank 210 mL milkshake + 10 ounces water + 5 ounces broth + 6 ounces punch.

_____

Calculate the total fluid output for each patient. If the patient was incontinent, denote each episode with an X and the number of incontinent episodes (Incontinent once = X1, Incontinent twice = X2, Incontinent three times = X3, etc.).

7. Mr. Lieberman was incontinent of urine one time on your shift. He voided 3 times in the urinal as follows: 8:00 AM—incontinent; 10:30 AM—voided 215 mL; 1:00 PM—voided 190 mL; 2:50 PM—voided 285 mL

8. Miss Romcevich voided 3 times as follows: 7:15 AM—325 mL, 10:10 AM—390 mL; 1:50 PM—285 mL.

9. Mrs. Lewis voided 5 times as follows: 7:40 AM—220 mL; 9:15 AM—190 mL; 11:50 AM—260 mL; 1:10 PM—205 mL; 2:30 PM—170 mL.

10. Mr. Beaugee vomited 250 mL at 7:55 AM. He voided twice as follows: 340 mL at 10:00 AM and 280 mL at 1:45 PM.

11. Mrs. Hernandez had a large, involuntary, liquid stool in bed at 7:10 AM. She voided 170 mL at 8:05 AM; 240 mL at 10:40 AM; 200 mL at 12:05 PM; and 265 mL at 2:35 PM.

12. Mr. Lim voided 310 mL at 7:15 AM; he was incontinent of a moderate amount at 10:00 AM; then voided 215 mL at 12:20 PM and voided 180 mL at 2:55 PM.

Gastrointestinal Elimination

OBJECTIVES

After completing this unit, you will be able to:

- Spell and define terms.
- Describe aging changes of the gastrointestinal system.
- Describe some common disorders of the gastrointestinal system.
- Describe nursing assistant actions related to the care of patients with disorders of the gastrointestinal system.
- List signs and symptoms the nursing assistant should observe for and report.
- Demonstrate Procedures 72–77 (set out in this unit in the textbook).

UNIT SUMMARY

The organs in the digestive system are very complex. Because of their complexity, disease of these organs is fairly common. Common conditions include:

- Hernias
- Inflammation such as cholecystitis
- Cancer
- Ulcerations

Procedures performed on this system include:

- Enemas (enemas are also performed before surgery on other parts of the body)

- Insertion of rectal tubes to relieve flatus
- Insertion of rectal suppositories

Great care must be exercised when performing these procedures. Remember that the patient's comfort and privacy should be protected at all times.

NURSING ASSISTANT ALERT

Action	Benefit
Provide adequate coverage and privacy.	Diminishes patient anxiety and embarrassment.
Maintain a matter-of-fact attitude.	Protects patient's self-esteem.
Prepare patients for tests according to orders.	Ensures more successful testing.

ACTIVITIES

Vocabulary Exercise

Complete the word search puzzle using the following clues. Write the name of the missing word on the line of each clue.

s	s	s	i	s	l	a	t	s	i	r	e	p	u	y
s	i	t	y	k	v	w	y	y	b	e	l	r	m	s
y	i	t	o	k	l	l	o	s	t	o	g	o	c	i
r	d	s	i	m	v	d	z	p	o	e	t	p	o	t
o	i	p	a	l	a	k	g	t	n	c	y	r	l	i
t	a	m	t	i	o	f	s	c	e	h	e	o	o	l
i	r	u	h	d	h	c	y	t	v	b	y	l	s	u
s	r	q	g	c	x	t	s	w	k	f	v	a	t	c
o	h	n	b	b	b	y	i	f	n	h	r	p	o	i
p	e	z	n	a	c	f	k	l	i	y	n	s	m	t
p	a	h	m	e	c	r	n	d	e	a	p	e	y	r
u	r	e	l	w	y	u	p	w	n	l	t	o	b	e
s	n	o	m	y	b	m	f	v	u	m	o	u	w	v
e	h	k	n	o	i	t	c	a	p	m	i	h	s	i
c	n	o	i	t	a	p	i	t	s	n	o	c	c	d

1. Gallbladder removal _____

2. Gallstones _____

3. Inflammation of small sacs in the colon _____

4. Difficulty in defecating _____

5. Wavelike movement that propels solid wastes through the intestinal tract _____

6. Medication used to help the bowels eliminate feces _____

7. An artificial opening in the abdomen for the purpose of evacuation of feces _____

8. The most serious form of constipation, in which stool is retained in the rectum, where water is absorbed

_____

9. Multiple loose stools _____

10. A condition that occurs when a large portion of the rectum protrudes from the body

_____

11. A person with ulcerative _____ will have multiple, foul-smelling, watery stools

12. Need to eliminate _____

13. Intestinal gas _____

14. Injection of fluid into the rectum to remove stool _____

15. Artificial opening for a colostomy _____

16. Solid body waste _____

Completion

Complete the following statements in the spaces provided.

1. Identify the equipment pictured.

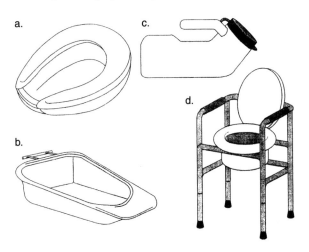

a. _____

b. _____

c. _____

d. _____

2. Carefully study the picture below and identify the barriers to aiding the patient's normal elimination pattern.

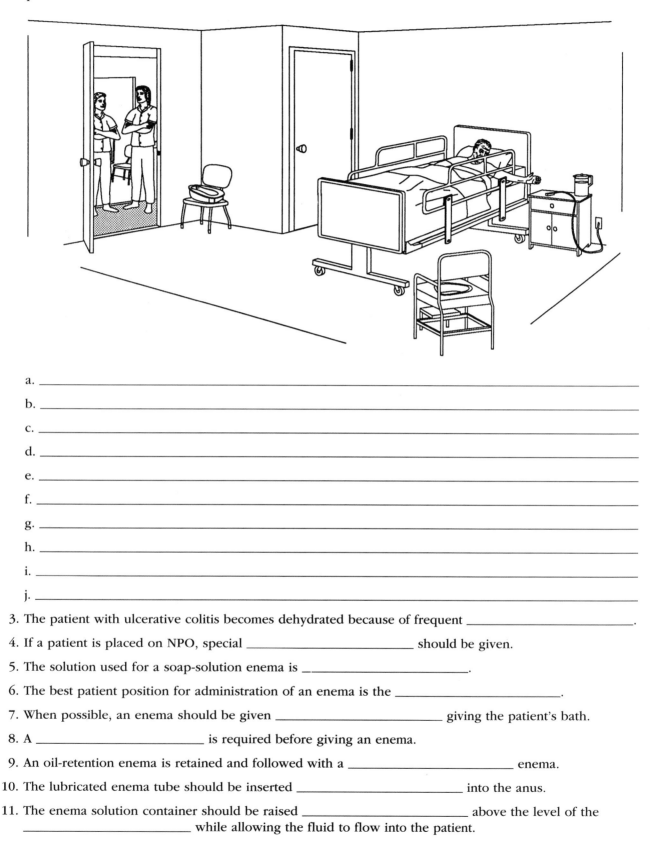

a. _____

b. _____

c. _____

d. _____

e. _____

f. _____

g. _____

h. _____

i. _____

j. _____

3. The patient with ulcerative colitis becomes dehydrated because of frequent _____.

4. If a patient is placed on NPO, special _____ should be given.

5. The solution used for a soap-solution enema is _____.

6. The best patient position for administration of an enema is the _____.

7. When possible, an enema should be given _____ giving the patient's bath.

8. A _____ is required before giving an enema.

9. An oil-retention enema is retained and followed with a _____ enema.

10. The lubricated enema tube should be inserted _____ into the anus.

11. The enema solution container should be raised _____ above the level of the _____ while allowing the fluid to flow into the patient.

12. Reusable enema equipment should be rinsed in _____ water before washing.

13. The rectal tube is used to relieve abdominal _____.

14. Commercially prepared chemical enema solutions drain fluid from the body to stimulate _____.

15. The chemical enema solution should be retained as _____.

16. Rectal tubes should be used no more than _____ in 24 hours.

17. Standard precautions require the use of _____ to protect the _____ from contamination during procedures involving the anus or rectum.

18. List five reasons that enemas are commonly given.

   a. _____

   b. _____

   c. _____

   d. _____

   e. _____

19. What information should be included when documenting an enema?

   a. _____

   b. _____

   c. _____

   d. _____

Clinical Situations

Briefly describe how a nursing assistant should react to the following situations.

1. You have an order to give a soap-solution enema and the patient has just finished breakfast.

   _____

2. The patient complains of cramping while you are giving an enema.

   _____

   _____

3. Your patient expresses concern about retaining a rectal suppository.

   _____

   _____

RELATING TO THE NURSING PROCESS

Write the step of the nursing process that is related to the nursing assistant action.

Nursing Assistant Action	Nursing Process Step
1. The nursing assistant carefully explains the procedure before administering an enema to the patient.	_____
2. The nursing assistant inserts a lubricating suppository beyond the rectal sphincter.	_____
3. The nursing assistant instructs the patient that an oil-retention enema must be retained for at least 20 minutes after introduction.	_____
4. The nursing assistant lubricates the tip of the enema tube well before insertion.	_____
5. The nursing assistant reports and records the results of the soap-solution enema.	_____
6. The nursing assistant plans her schedule so she can give an enema before breakfast. She plans to bathe the patient after the procedure.	_____
7. The nursing assistant notes an abnormality in the enema returns. She saves the stool for the nurse to inspect, and informs the nurse of the problem.	_____

DEVELOPING GREATER INSIGHT

Answer the questions below based upon the following situation.

Mrs. Lebowitz is a 79-year-old cognitively impaired patient. You have not cared for this patient in a week. The previous shift did not report any problems with the patient. She felt warm, so you checked her temperature. She has a fever of 101.8°F (R). She has been sleeping more than usual. She keeps falling asleep in her chair, which is out of character for the patient. She frequently rubs her lower abdomen, which is slightly distended. She has had two small, incontinent, liquid stools today. This is unusual. You have been assigned to administer enemas to this patient in the past because she tends to be constipated. She has been passing gas. She has voided 4 times during the first 4 hours of your shift. Each time, she was incontinent a small amount of urine. Normally, she eats 100% of her meals, but today she is refusing to eat. She is taking liquids, but has complained of nausea. When you get the flow sheet book to document her liquid stools, you notice that she has not had a BM in 3 days. Four days ago she had a small BM. She had a small BM five days ago. She had no BM on day 6 or 7. She had a small BM on day 8. You see that her appetite has decreased over the past few days.

1. What action will you take?

   _____

   _____

2. What is the most likely cause of the patient's problem?

   _____

   _____

3. Why does liquid stool suggest a problem?

   _____

   _____

4. Does this situation require immediate action, or will you report your observations at the end of the shift?

   _____

   _____

Nutritional Needs and Diet Modifications

OBJECTIVES

After completing this unit, you will be able to:

- Spell and define terms.
- Define normal nutrition.
- List the essential nutrients.
- Name the six groups listed on the food pyramid.
- Identify the basic facility diets and describe each.
- State the purpose of calorie counts and food intake studies.
- Describe general care for the patient with dysphagia and swallowing problems.
- List types of alternative nutrition.
- Demonstrate Procedures 78 and 79 (set out in this unit in the textbook).

UNIT SUMMARY

The six nutrients essential to health are:

- Proteins
- Carbohydrates
- Fats
- Vitamins
- Minerals
- Water

Food is usually taken into the body through the mouth. Sometimes, however, alternative ways of meeting dietary needs must be found. For example:

- Enteral feeding
- Hyperalimentation

Nutritional needs are best met when selections are made properly from the food guide pyramid:

- Meat and beans
- Dairy

- Vegetables
- Fruits
- Breads, cereals, and pastas (grains)
- Oils

Foods for hospital diets are selected from the food guide pyramid. They are prepared in special ways. There are four routine hospital diets:

- House, regular, general, or select
- Liquid, clear
- Liquid, full
- Soft

Many special or therapeutic diets are also prescribed. The patient's dietary intake is based on:

- Personal preference
- Health requirements
- Religious preferences

Calorie counts and food intake studies may be done to determine the nutritional adequacy and caloric content of the patient's diet.

Patients with dysphagia have difficulty swallowing food and fluids and are at high risk of aspiration.

Fluid intake and output must be carefully balanced for good health:

- Fluids are measured in milliliters (mL) or cubic centimeters (cc).
- Fluids come from and are lost through multiple sources.
- Fluid intake and output must be accurately measured and recorded when ordered.

The nursing assistant helps meet the patient's nutritional needs by:

- Serving trays
- Serving special nourishments
- Providing fresh drinking water
- Assisting patients with feeding
- Feeding patients who are unable to feed themselves
- Assisting patients who have swallowing problems

NURSING ASSISTANT ALERT

Action	Benefit
Check diet against patient identification.	Ensures that correct patient gets proper nutrition.
Present food attractively.	Encourages appetite.
Serve food at the proper temperature.	Prevents foodborne illness and improves patient acceptance of foods.
Follow all infection control precautions.	Prevents the spread of infection and avoids cross-contamination.
Use an unhurried attitude.	Decreases the risk of aspiration. Patients improve consumption when not rushed.
Follow orders regarding food or fluid restrictions.	Restrictions are part of the therapy for many conditions.
Position patients for meals.	Ensures comfort, prevents choking, and maximizes the patient's ability to feed self.
Assist patients as needed by opening packages, preparing tray, cutting meat, feeding, or assisting/encouraging to eat, as needed.	Ensures that food is prepared so the patient can eat it readily. If the patient needs assistance, ensures that food is served at the correct temperature and needed help is received.
Accurately document food intake.	Creates a record of calories and nutrients consumed for dietitian and physician evaluation.
Measure intake and output carefully.	Contributes to accurate evaluation.

ACTIVITIES

Vocabulary Exercise

Complete the puzzle by filling in the missing letters of the words found in this unit. Use the definitions to help you discover these words.

1.   N _ _ _ _ _ _ _ _   1. The process by which the body uses food for growth and repair

2.   _ _ _ _ U _ _ _ _   2. Supplies roughage

3.   _ _ _ _ _ _ T _ _ _   3. Elimination of solid wastes

4. _ _ _ _ _ _ _ _ R _ _ _ _   4. Energy foods

5.   _ _ _ _ _ _ I _ _   5. Process of breaking down food into simple substances that can be used for nourishment

6.   _ _ _ _ E _ _   6. Nutrient used for building and repair

7.   _ _ N _ _ _ _ _   7. Inorganic chemical nutrients that help build body tissues and regulate the chemistry of body fluids

8.   _ _ T _ _ _ _ _   8. Nutrients necessary for normal metabolism

9.   _ _ _ S   9. Nutrients used to store energy

Completion

Complete the following statements in the spaces provided.

1. TPN, which stands for _____, is an intravenous solution.

2. Carbohydrates and fats are called _____ foods because the body uses them to produce heat and energy.

3. Proteins are composed of _____ acids.

4. Complete proteins contain all the amino acids that the body _____ manufacture.

5. When a postoperative patient tolerates the diet at one level, he or she is _____.

6. The first postoperative intake usually permitted is _____ or sips of water.

7. The clear liquid diet does not irritate the bowel or encourage _____.

8. If a patient is on I&O and you serve him nourishments, you must _____ _____.

9. Before serving a tray, be sure to clear away anything that is _____ _____.

10. When feeding a helpless patient, hold the spoon at a _____ to the patient's mouth.

11. Nutritional supplements are ordered by the physician and have _____.

12. A mechanically altered diet may be served to patients who have problems _____ or _____.

13. A pureed diet is commonly served to patients who have difficulty _____.

14. When a patient has an order for a calorie count, all food intake is accurately _____ at the end of each meal.

15. Patients with _____ have difficulty swallowing fluids and food and are at high risk of aspiration.

16. The speech language pathologist may order addition of _____ to liquids for patients who have swallowing problems.

17. Sodium-restricted diets are some of the _____ diets for patients to follow.

True/False

Mark the following true or false by circling T or F.

1.   T   F   Patients who are unable to swallow without aspiration may require alternative nutrition.

2.   T   F   TPN is a technique that introduces nutrients into a vein.

3.   T   F   Enteral feedings are introduced into smaller veins in the arm.

4.   T   F   Gastrostomy feedings enter the stomach through a nasogastric tube.

5.   T   F   Enteral feedings are usually controlled by an automatic device.

6.   T   F   Oral hygiene may safely be omitted when patients receive enteral feedings, because food does not enter the mouth.

7.   T   F   Nausea or vomiting must be reported immediately to the nurse.

8.   T   F   The head of the bed should be flat during feedings and remain in that position for half an hour after completion of the feeding.

9.   T   F   Patients must not be permitted to lie on enteral tubes.

10.   T   F   Liquid nutritional supplements should be served at mealtime.

11.   T   F   Completing a food intake or calorie count study requires a team effort.

12.   T   F   Patients with dysphagia are at high risk of developing malnutrition and dehydration.

Short Answer

Briefly answer the following questions.

1. What are the names of three health care facility diets?

   a. _____

   b. _____

   c. _____

2. Why is an unhurried attitude important when feeding a patient?

   _____

3. Name two alternative methods of providing nutrients.

   a. _____

   b. _____

4. Three functions of nutrients are:

   a. _____

   b. _____

   c. _____

5. The six basic nutrients are:

    a. _____

    b. _____

    c. _____

    d. _____

    e. _____

    f. _____

6. Six minerals needed in any person's daily diet include:

    a. _____

    b. _____

    c. _____

    d. _____

    e. _____

    f. _____

7. Two functions of vitamins are to:

    a. _____

    b. _____

8. Six vitamins needed by the body are:

    a. _____

    b. _____

    c. _____

    d. _____

    e. _____

    f. _____

9. Name five foods to be avoided in a low-sodium diet.

    a. _____

    b. _____

    c. _____

    d. _____

    e. _____

10. The total daily intake from the following food groups is:

    a. fruit _____

    b. vegetables _____

    c. meat _____

    d. grains _____

11. What is the purpose of serving nutritional supplements?

    _____

    _____

12. Explain the difference between supplements and nourishments.

_____

_____

_____

_____

13. Hot foods must be served at _____°F or above, and cold foods must be served at _____ °F or below.

14. Explain why the food cart must be separated from the soiled linen hamper and housekeeping cart by at least one room's width in the hallways.

_____

_____

_____

_____

15. List three things you can do to maintain food temperature when the food cart arrives on the unit.

a. _____

b. _____

c. _____

16. Explain the difference between a PEG tube and a nasogastric tube, and state the purpose of each tube.

_____

_____

Matching

Identify the type of vitamin.

1. vitamin A _____

2. vitamin B complex _____

3. vitamin C _____

4. vitamin D _____

5. vitamin E _____

6. vitamin K _____

a. water-soluble

b. fat-soluble

Classification

Complete the chart in the spaces provided.

1. Write the names of the six food guide pyramid categories at the top of the columns below. Write the names of each of the following foods in the column under the proper food group.

apples	bacon	beef	bread	butter	cereal
cheese	chicken	cottage cheese	fish	flour	honey
ice cream	liver	milk	olive oil	pasta	pears
peas	rice	spinach	yogurt		

Group 1	Group 2	Group 3	Group 4	Group 5	Group 6
_____	_____	_____	_____	_____	_____
_____	_____	_____	_____	_____	_____
_____	_____	_____	_____	_____	_____
_____	_____	_____	_____	_____	_____
_____	_____	_____	_____	_____	_____

Clinical Situations

Briefly describe how a nursing assistant should react to the following situations.

1. Your patient is on I&O and you picked up the lunch tray.

_____

2. You serve a tray to a blind person who is able to feed himself.

_____

3. Your patient's chart includes an order to force fluids.

_____

4. The patient receiving an IV has 25 mL of fluid left in the bag.

_____

5. Your patient is on a strict kosher diet and the tray has a shrimp salad as an entree.

_____

Conversions

Convert the following values into milliliters. Show your work.

1. 2 (8-oz) cups of coffee _____ _____ mL

2. 1 (6-oz) bowl of soup _____ _____ mL

3. 3 (8-oz) glasses of water _____ _____ mL

4. 2 (4-oz) glasses of ice chips _____ _____ mL

5. 2 (4-oz) dishes of gelatin _____ _____ mL

Completion

1. Keep a diary of your food intake for 24 hours. Include everything you eat. Then answer the following questions to determine if you achieved an adequate intake of nutrients.

Dietary Chart

Time	Food	Amount

Answer the following questions by entering Yes or No in the space provided.

_____ Did you include the recommended number of servings from the meat group?

_____ Did you include the recommended number of servings from the bread, cereal, rice, and pasta group?

_____ Did you include the recommended amount of milk or its equivalent in dairy products?

_____ Did you include at least 1 serving of a food high in vitamin C?

_____ Did you make sure there was some roughage in your diet?

_____ Did you include the recommended number of servings from the vegetable group?

_____ Are there things in your diet that you think should be eliminated?

2. Complete the food pyramid by writing the correct word(s) or number(s) on the spaces provided.

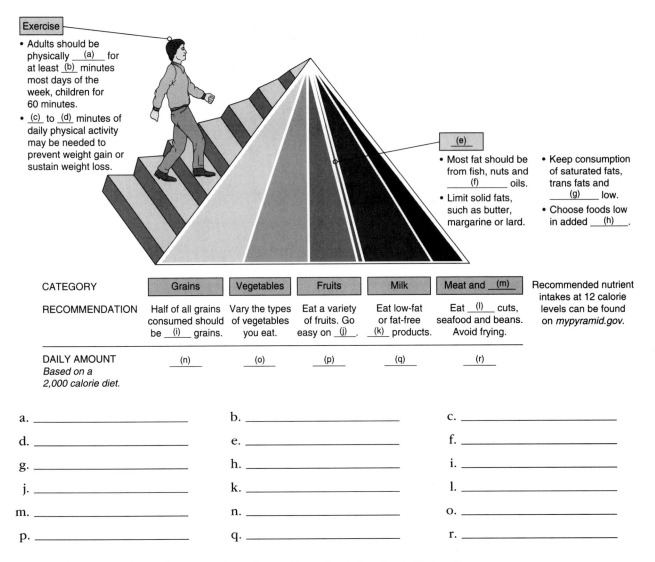

Exercise
- Adults should be physically __(a)__ for at least __(b)__ minutes most days of the week, children for 60 minutes.
- __(c)__ to __(d)__ minutes of daily physical activity may be needed to prevent weight gain or sustain weight loss.

(e)
- Most fat should be from fish, nuts and __(f)__ oils.
- Limit solid fats, such as butter, margarine or lard.
- Keep consumption of saturated fats, trans fats and __(g)__ low.
- Choose foods low in added __(h)__.

CATEGORY	Grains	Vegetables	Fruits	Milk	Meat and __(m)__	Recommended nutrient intakes at 12 calorie levels can be found on *mypyramid.gov*.
RECOMMENDATION	Half of all grains consumed should be __(i)__ grains.	Vary the types of vegetables you eat.	Eat a variety of fruits. Go easy on __(j)__.	Eat low-fat or fat-free __(k)__ products.	Eat __(l)__ cuts, seafood and beans. Avoid frying.	
DAILY AMOUNT *Based on a 2,000 calorie diet.*	__(n)__	__(o)__	__(p)__	__(q)__	__(r)__	

a. _____   b. _____   c. _____

d. _____   e. _____   f. _____

g. _____   h. _____   i. _____

j. _____   k. _____   l. _____

m. _____   n. _____   o. _____

p. _____   q. _____   r. _____

3. Complete an intake and output sheet that reflects the following information.

The patient, John Rodriquez, is in Room 404B. During the day he felt fairly well. He drank about 50 mL of water after he brushed his teeth at 0715. He also voided 550 mL of yellow urine. Breakfast arrived and he had a pot of tea (240 mL). Early-morning nourishments arrived and he selected and consumed 120 mL of cranberry juice followed by 80 mL of water at lunch (1115), with 120 mL of orange sherbet for dessert. He voided again, 400 mL yellow urine, at 1430. During the afternoon he had 240 mL of tea with a visitor. Dinner arrived and he had 180 mL of milk, 180 mL of soup, and 120 mL of gelatin. He asked for a urinal and voided 375 mL of urine. At 2130 he tried to eat some gelatin, approximately 50 mL, and within minutes vomited 400 mL. He continued to feel nauseated and vomited 200 mL at 2315, 150 mL at 2400, and 80 mL at 0230. At 0530, 500 mL D/W were started IV. Mr. Rodriquez voided 300 mL at this time. The urine was pink-tinged.

WASHINGTON GENERAL HOSPITAL
FLUID INTAKE AND OUTPUT

Name _____ Room _____

Date	Time	Method of Adm.	Intake			Output		
			Solution	Amounts Rec'd	Time	Urine Amount	Others Kind	Amount
Total								

RELATING TO THE NURSING PROCESS

Write the step of the nursing process that is related to the nursing assistant action.

Nursing Assistant Action   **Nursing Process Step**

1. The nursing assistant carefully checks the patient's identification band against the tray tag.

   _____

2. The nursing assistant reports to the nurse that the patient ate only one-third of the soft diet ordered.

   _____

3. The nursing assistant documents that the patient refused lunch because he felt nauseated.

   _____

4. The nursing assistant carefully records the fluids taken by the patient who has an order for I&O.

   _____

5. The nursing assistant checks with the team leader to be sure gelatin should be recorded as fluid intake.

   _____

6. The nursing assistant makes a special note during report that her patient is on I&O.

   _____

DEVELOPING GREATER INSIGHT

Mrs. Gillaspie was hospitalized and diagnosed with dehydration. The dietitian noted that she was underweight, with laboratory values suggesting malnutrition. The dehydration was corrected with a combination of oral fluids and IVs. The nurse informs you that it will take several months to correct the malnutrition. The physician discussed the need for a gastrostomy feeding tube with the patient and family. They decided to delay the procedure and to return the patient to the long-term care facility and try to work on her weight.

Mrs. Gillaspie is a very picky eater. The physician ordered daily weights and oral nutritional supplements at 10:00 AM, 4:00 PM, and 9:00 PM. You notice that the patient likes the supplements, but they are sweet and filling, and if the patient drinks the supplement, she does not eat her meals. She likes sweet beverages better than water, but will drink water if it is very cold with a lot of ice.

You also notice that Mrs. Gillaspie often eats a little of the food on her meal tray, then hoards other food items in her room to eat later. Unfortunately, she often forgets to eat them, and you have had to throw spoiled and moldy food items away because they were not refrigerated. One day you found her eating pudding that she had hoarded from her lunch tray two days ago. You informed the nurse, because the milk-based pudding had not been refrigerated or covered. Now you check the room after each meal and remove potentially unsafe items. If you refrigerate an item in the unit pantry, and offer it to her later, the patient usually accepts it. Otherwise she forgets about the refrigerated items.

The patient will eat in between meals if she likes the food. She particularly likes fruit. She dislikes meats that are difficult to chew, and dark green vegetables such as spinach and broccoli. She will eat breads if prepared with jelly or honey, but will not eat buttered bread, biscuits, or rolls.

Mrs. Gillaspie's family plans to return her to the long-term care facility, but the physician and dietitian are concerned that her malnutrition will worsen and that the dehydration will recur. The nurse informs you that personnel from the long-term care facility, the dietitian, staff from your unit, and the patient's family will be attending a care plan meeting at 2:00 PM to address the patient's nutritional needs. She asks you to attend the meeting because you know the patient so well. What information will you share and/or suggest to help the team develop a care plan for this patient?

_____

_____

_____

_____

_____

_____

_____

_____

_____

_____

Caring for Patients with Special Needs

Caring for the Perioperative Patient

OBJECTIVES

After completing this unit, you will be able to:

- Spell and define terms.
- Describe the concerns of patients who are about to have surgery.
- Identify the three main components of perioperative care and list the nursing assistant responsibilities for each.
- Describe nursing assistant actions and observations related to the care of perioperative patients.
- Prepare the unit for the patient's return from the operating room.
- Give routine postoperative care.
- Recognize reportable observations of patients in the postoperative period.
- Assist the patient with deep breathing and coughing.
- Identify nursing assistant responsibilities in the care of patients with wounds and drains.
- Apply elasticized stockings and pneumatic hosiery.
- Describe the effects of heat and cold applications.
- Demonstrate Procedures 80–84 (set out in this unit in the textbook).

UNIT SUMMARY

Perioperative care is given to patients before, during, and after surgery.

The surgical patient requires continuous care before, during, and after surgery. The nursing assistant helps in preoperative and postoperative care.

Nursing assistant responsibilities in the preoperative period include:

- Preparing the operative site
- Readying the patient on the morning of surgery
- Helping transfer the patient to and from the stretcher
- Providing emotional support

Nursing assistant responsibilities during the operative period include:

- Preparing a surgical (postoperative) bed
- Securing and setting up equipment needed for the postoperative period

Nursing assistant responsibilities in the postoperative period include:

- Assisting in the transfer from stretcher to bed
- Carefully observing and reporting

- Monitoring vital signs frequently, as directed by the nurse or according to facility policy
- Assisting the patient with postoperative exercises, including:
  o Position changes
  o Leg exercises
  o Respiratory exercises
- Applying elasticized stockings and pneumatic hosiery
- Assisting in dangling and initial ambulation
- Using standard precautions whenever contact with blood, body fluids, secretions, excretions, mucous membranes, or nonintact skin is likely
- Monitoring dressings, wounds, and drains, and assisting in the care of these items, as permitted by facility policy

NURSING ASSISTANT ALERT

Action	Benefit
Provide emotional support by being calm, efficient, and a willing listener.	Builds patient confidence and helps reduce fears.
Carry out pre- and postoperative orders carefully.	Reduces the likelihood of postoperative complications.
Assemble necessary equipment and conscientiously prepare the patient's room for the return from surgery.	Appropriate care can be given immediately. Time is not wasted.
Observe the patient closely as postoperative exercise and ambulation are attempted. Be prepared to assist.	Avoids patient injury and prevents complications.
Report observations accurately and promptly.	Suggests and enables nursing interventions to promote recovery. Keeps nurse informed of patient's status.

ACTIVITIES

Vocabulary Exercise

Complete the puzzle by filling in the missing letters of words found in this unit. Use the definitions to help you discover these words.

1. _ _ _ _ _ _ _ S _ _   1. artificial body part
2.   _ _ _ U _ _ _ _ _ _   2. walking
3.   _ _ R _ _ _ _ _   3. dizziness
4.   _ _ _ G _ _ _ _ _   4. hiccup
5.   _ _ _ _ _ I _ _   5. sitting with feet over bed edge
6.   _ _ _ _ C _ _ _ _ _ 6. infection that develops in the hospital
7. _ _ _ _ _ _ _ A _ _ _   7. collapse of lung tissue
8.   _ _ _ _ L _ _   8. a clot that breaks off and travels through the vascular system

Matching

Match each statement on the left with the correct word on the right.

1. _____ opening into the body   a. embolus

2. _____ the period following surgery   b. dyspnea

3. _____ drawing foreign material into the lungs   c. pallor

4. _____ lack of adequate oxygen supply   d. singultus

5. _____ loss of feeling or sensation   e. orifice

6. _____ inflammation of veins that can cause blood clots   f. vertigo

7. _____ dizziness   g. thrombophlebitis

8. _____ less than normal skin color   h. postoperative

9. _____ difficulty breathing   i. hypoxia

10. _____ moving blood clot   j. aspiration

                                                                           k. anesthesia

Completion

Complete the following statements in the spaces provided.

1. The three phases of care required by the surgical patient are:

   a. _____

   b. _____

   c. _____

2. The purpose of anesthesia is _____.

3. Anesthetics _____ body temperature.

4. When patients have general anesthesia, they are apt to become nauseated and may _____ postoperatively.

5. With a local anesthetic, the patient may remain _____ during surgery.

6. When a spinal anesthetic is given, all sensations _____ the level of the injection are _____.

7. Seven duties the nursing assistant may be assigned in regard to the preoperative patient are:

   a. _____

   b. _____

   c. _____

   d. _____

   e. _____

   f. _____

   g. _____

8. Equipment left on the bedside table after the recovery bed is made includes:

   _____

9. When a patient vomits, his head should be _____ to prevent _____.

10. Patient questions should be referred to the _____.

11. The patient's position should be changed every _____ hours following surgery.

12. Before ambulating, assist the patient to _____ at the bedside.

13. Binders that are ordered postoperatively must be:

    a. _____

    b. _____

    c. _____

14. Elasticized stockings are applied postoperatively to help support the _____ of the legs.

15. Postoperative leg exercises should be performed _____ times every _____ hours.

Complete the following statements regarding postoperative discomfort.

16. The patient complains of thirst. You should give special _____ care and check for signs of _____.

17. The patient who had her gallbladder removed has singultus. You should support the _____ area.

18. The patient complains of pain. You should report the _____, _____, and _____ of pain.

19. The patient's abdomen is distended. You should encourage increased _____.

20. The patient has urinary retention. You should monitor _____ carefully.

21. The patient is hemorrhaging. You should keep the patient quiet and check _____.

22. The patient may be going into shock. You suspect this because there is a fall in _____, the pulse is _____, the skin is _____, and the skin color is pale.

23. The patient is suffering from hypoxia. You should _____ to a sitting or _____ position and monitor oxygen if ordered.

24. The patient has suffered wound disruption. You should keep the patient _____ and _____ the incision area.

25. A _____ is used to apply heat or cold to a specific area of the body.

26. A _____ is used to apply heat or cold to the patient's entire body.

27. Heat applications _____ the blood vessels.

28. Cold applications _____ the blood vessels.

29. List three reasons for using local cold applications.

    a. _____

    b. _____

    c. _____

Surgical Prep Areas

Using a colored pencil or crayon, shade in the surgical prep areas that are to be shaved before the indicated surgery.

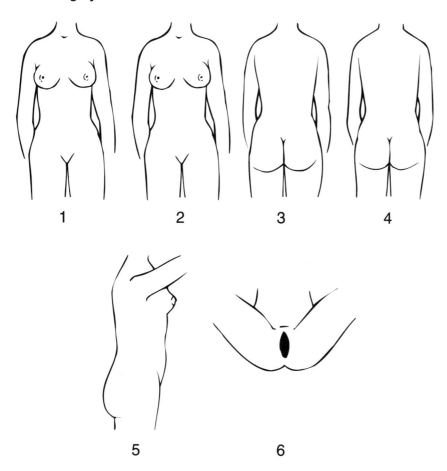

1. abdominal surgery

2. breast surgery—anterior

3. breast surgery—posterior

4. back surgery

5. kidney surgery

6. vaginal, rectal, and perineal surgery

Short Answer

Answer the following questions.

1. What actions should you take after the preoperative medication is given?

    a. _____

    b. _____

    c. _____

    d. _____

    e. _____

2. What actions would you take while the patient is in the operating room?

    a. _____

    b. _____

    c. _____

3. What actions should be taken when the patient returns from surgery?

    a. _____

    b. _____

    c. _____

    d. _____

    e. _____

4. What special precautions should be taken when drainage tubes are in place?

    a. _____

    b. _____

    c. _____

    d. _____

    e. _____

    f. _____

    g. _____

    h. _____

5. Examine the following surgical checklist. List the items that are direct nursing assistant responsibilities.

    a. _____

    b. _____

    c. _____

    d. _____

    e. _____

    f. _____

    g. _____

    h. _____

    i. _____

1. Admission sheet

2. Surgical consent

3. Sterilization consent (if necessary)

4. Consultation sheet (if necessary)

5. History and physical

6. Lab reports (pregnancy tests also, if necessary)

7. Surgery prep done and charted, if required

8. Latest TPR and blood pressure charted

9. Preoperative medication given and charted (if required)

10. Wrist identification band on patient

11. Fingernail polish and makeup removed

12. Metallic objects removed (rings may be taped)

13. Dentures removed

14. Other prostheses removed (such as artificial limb or eye)

15. Bath blanket and head cap in place

16. Bed in high position and side rails up after preop medication is given

17. Patient has voided

6. Describe how to determine which size of anti-embolism hosiery should be used for the patient and explain why having the correct size is important.

_____

_____

_____

_____

True/False

Mark the following true or false by circling T or F.

1. T F Vital signs should be taken every 2 hours during the immediate postoperative period.

2. T F In most facilities, pain is considered to be the fifth vital sign.

3. T F Bandages are used to cover the wound.

4. T F Dressings are wrapped around bandages to hold them in place.

5. T F Montgomery straps are long adhesive strips with ties to hold dressings in place.

6. T F Sequential compression therapy is used to prevent blood clots.

7. T F Check the brachial and femoral pulses before applying pneumatic hosiery.

8. T F Pneumatic hosiery may be applied over anti-embolism hose.

9. T F Pneumatic hosiery should be removed every 6 hours for 30 minutes.

10. T F Deep vein thrombosis and pulmonary embolus (blood clot in the lungs) are serious postoperative complications.

11. T F Binders may be used to hold dressings in place.

Clinical Situations

Briefly describe how a nursing assistant should react to the following situations.

1. You are assisting a patient with initial ambulation, and the patient faints.

_____

_____

2. You find that the anti-embolism stockings your patient is wearing are wrinkled and have slipped down his leg.

_____

_____

3. Your postoperative patient's blood pressure has dropped and her pulse is rapid and weak. Her skin is cold and moist.

_____

_____

4. Your postoperative patient is anxious, has a feeling of heaviness in his chest, and is cyanotic.

_____

_____

RELATING TO THE NURSING PROCESS

Write the step of the nursing process that is related to the nursing assistant action.

Nursing Assistant Action	Nursing Process Step
1. The nursing assistant listens to and reports to the nurse the patient's concerns about scheduled surgery.	_____
2. The nursing assistant helps the patient bathe or shower with surgical soap.	_____
3. The nursing assistant checks with the nurse to determine the specific area to be shaved for surgery.	_____
4. Following shaving, the nursing assistant removes unattached hairs by gently pressing the sticky side of surgical tape against them.	_____
5. The nursing assistant makes sure there are no wrinkles in elasticized stockings once they are applied.	_____
6. The nursing assistant finds that the patient's pulse rate has increased more than 10 bpm after initial standing. The nursing assistant returns the patient to bed and reports to the nurse.	_____

Caring for the Emotionally Stressed Patient

OBJECTIVES

After completing this unit, you will be able to:

- Spell and define terms.
- Define mental health.
- Explain how physical and mental health are related.
- Identify common mental health problems.
- Describe nursing assistant actions and observations related to the care of patients with mental health needs.
- Describe ways of helping patients cope with stressful situations.
- Identify professional boundaries in relationships with patients and families.

UNIT SUMMARY

Mental and physical health are interrelated. They influence the individual's ability to cope with life within the framework of society.

Failure of coping mechanisms leads to maladaptive behaviors. The nursing assistant has specific responsibilities when caring for patients who exhibit maladaptive behaviors. These include:

- Observing and objectively reporting behaviors
- Ensuring patient safety

- Intervening in behaviors as directed by the care plan
- Respecting professional boundaries with patients and families
- Behaving in an ethical manner and avoiding personal relationships with patients and families

NURSING ASSISTANT ALERT

Action	Benefit
Observe and objectively report patient behaviors.	Ensures correct evaluation.
Closely supervise patient activities.	Prevents patient injury.
Use consistency in your approach.	Helps patients reorient. Lessens the degree of confusion. Contributes to patient's sense of security.
Be vigilant in recognizing potentially unsafe situations.	Allows early interventions that reduce the likelihood of injury to patients or staff.

ACTIVITIES

Vocabulary Exercise

In the puzzle, find and circle each of the following words. In the space provided, define each word.

a	D	p	a	s	r	e	p	r	e	s	s	i	o	n	m	y	T	s	d
d	c	A	a	n	i	o	b	s	e	s	s	i	o	n	g	y	u	i	y
a	o	C	S	r	o	s	h	O	V	G	W	R	M	D	X	i	s	t	d
p	m	b	a	a	a	r	a	G	B	e	c	T	z	T	c	o	e	e	B
t	p	l	g	s	i	n	e	i	r	K	Y	W	u	i	r	i	n	z	d
a	u	V	i	t	G	b	o	x	r	n	e	Q	d	i	x	i	j	y	v
t	l	O	t	r	w	p	o	i	i	d	r	e	e	n	a	g	F	A	k
i	s	n	a	e	Y	c	U	h	a	a	n	n	a	l	l	W	y	R	s
o	i	o	t	s	r	e	W	u	p	R	t	o	e	H	R	A	G	l	n
n	o	i	i	s	Y	q	X	e	f	a	s	n	h	Z	E	C	s	F	o
W	n	t	o	o	O	l	e	O	t	u	a	D	a	c	W	l	t	Z	i
G	k	c	n	r	z	a	w	i	p	b	y	T	C	i	o	X	u	M	s
j	o	e	c	s	z	G	o	p	l	U	x	S	a	g	m	p	p	l	u
H	x	j	y	G	Y	n	r	i	u	Y	O	S	D	p	n	i	y	i	l
s	o	o	o	s	p	e	n	s	k	h	C	w	p	F	l	i	l	h	e
o	Q	r	R	a	s	g	y	x	l	c	c	d	b	x	T	D	p	u	d
h	Y	p	n	s	Y	N	G	o	e	v	i	t	c	e	f	f	a	o	b
b	A	i	d	e	p	r	e	s	s	i	o	n	H	t	e	e	d	c
d	c	o	b	o	u	n	d	a	r	i	e	s	f	K	u	Y	J	a	Z
b	n	W	z	T	W	i	j	R	S	m	s	i	l	o	h	o	c	l	a

1. adaptation

_____

2. affective

_____

3. agitation

_____

4. alcoholism

_____

5. anorexia

_____

6. anxiety

_____

7. boundaries

_____

8. bulimia

_____

9. compulsion

_____

10. coping

_____

11. delusions

_____

12. depression

_____

13. disorientation

_____

14. DTs

_____

15. enabling

_____

16. obsession

_____

17. panic

_____

18. phobia

_____

19. SAD

_____

20. stressors

_____

21. suicide

_____

Completion

Complete the following statements in the spaces provided.

1. Mental health means exhibiting behaviors that reflect a person's _____ to the multiple stresses of life.

2. A situation that makes a person anxious about his well-being is called a _____.

3. Poor mental health is demonstrated by _____.

4. Physical and mental health are _____.

5. A word used to mean handling stress is _____ with stress.

6. People use _____ mechanisms to protect their self-esteem.

7. Demanding patients are usually only expressing their own _____.

8. Some people turn to alcohol as a means of _____.

9. Alcohol _____ brain activity.

10. Alcohol is a drug that mixes _____ with other drugs.

11. Older alcoholics have a _____ chance of recovery.

12. The best approach to the disoriented patient is one that is _____ and _____.

13. *Agitation* is defined as inappropriate vocal or _____ activity due to causes other than confusion or need.

14. The patient who is disoriented may benefit from _____ orientation.

15. An extreme maladaptive response in which the person feels everyone is against him is called _____.

16. The nursing assistant must be sensitive to non_____ clues to the sources of a patient's stress.

17. It is important for the patient who is under stress to feel that the nursing assistant is _____ and will respect privacy and feelings.

18. Be supportive of the patient's own _____ to overcome the stress.

19. Patients often show their frustrations by being very _____.

20. _____ are unspoken limits on physical and emotional relationships with patients.

21. You may be in a relationship _____ if you are being flirtatious with a patient.

22. _____ means reacting to a patient in a manner that shields the patient from experiencing the full impact or consequences of her actions or behavior.

True/False

Mark the following true or false by circling T or F.

1.	T	F	You can help patients cope with stress by being a good listener.
2.	T	F	You should try to make patients see situations from your point of view.
3.	T	F	If you know the patient is wrong, it is all right to argue the point.
4.	T	F	Panic attacks are mental illnesses involving anxiety reactions in response to stress.
5.	T	F	Disorientation and depression may be associated with both physical and mental disorders.
6.	T	F	The most common functional disorder in the geriatric age group is depression.
7.	T	F	Some properly used drugs can cause a person to feel depressed.
8.	T	F	A proper approach to the depressed patient is to let him know how sorry you feel for him.
9.	T	F	The person who threatens suicide never attempts it.
10.	T	F	An elderly person who has just lost a spouse is at risk for suicide.
11.	T	F	The suicidal patient needs help in restoring her feelings of self-esteem.
12.	T	F	Agitation is a significant problem for the elderly, their families, and the nursing staff.
13.	T	F	The patient who is agitated has a prolonged attention span.
14.	T	F	Constipation and dehydration can contribute to agitation.
15.	T	F	One way to help the depressed patient is to reinforce his self-concept as a valued member of society.
16.	T	F	The disoriented person may show disorientation to time, person, or place.
17.	T	F	Labeling a behavior implies passing judgment.
18.	T	F	Speaking to others in the same way the supervisor speaks to you is a form of compensation.
19.	T	F	OCD is one form of anxiety disorder.
20.	T	F	PTSD is commonly seen in survivors of major trauma.
21.	T	F	Panic attacks seldom recur.
22.	T	F	A compulsion is a thought that makes no sense.
23.	T	F	Phobias may cause a person to panic.
24.	T	F	Snakes, spiders, and rats are common triggers that cause a person to feel panic.
25.	T	F	Affective disorders are seldom characterized by a disturbance in mood.
26.	T	F	Patients with bipolar disorder have mood swings ranging from elation to severe depression.
27.	T	F	Schizoaffective disorder may be difficult to diagnose.
28.	T	F	Patients with borderline personality disorder are often very manipulative.
29.	T	F	Males do not develop eating disorders.
30.	T	F	Substance abuse may cause impaired judgment and maladaptive behavior.
31.	T	F	Culture affects a person's feelings about mental illness.
32.	T	F	The DTs usually occur when individuals withdraw from illegal drugs; they seldom occur as a result of use of substances such as alcohol, which can be legally purchased.
33.	T	F	Suicide precautions are measures and practices a facility follows if a patient is at risk of harming himself or herself.
34.	T	F	Suicide precautions are seldom necessary with persons who are mentally ill.
35.	T	F	Signs and symptoms of delirium tremens include hallucinations and tremors.

Short Answer

Briefly answer the following questions.

1. List four ways to deal successfully with a demanding patient.

   a. _____

   b. _____

   c. _____

   d. _____

2. List five nursing assistant approaches for caring for a patient who is depressed.

   a. _____

   b. _____

   c. _____

   d. _____

   e. _____

3. List eight signs and symptoms that suggest that a patient is contemplating suicide.

   a. _____

   b. _____

   c. _____

   d. _____

   e. _____

   f. _____

   g. _____

   h. _____

4. List six behaviors that suggest that a health care worker is crossing professional boundaries.

   a. _____

   b. _____

   c. _____

   d. _____

   e. _____

   f. _____

5. List six methods of assisting patients who have behavior problems.

   a. _____

   b. _____

   c. _____

   d. _____

   e. _____

   f. _____

Clinical Situations

Briefly describe how a nursing assistant should react to the following situations.

1. Mrs. Sears has trouble sleeping, seems lethargic, and frequently dabs tears from her eyes.

   _____

   _____

   _____

2. Mr. Osborn is recovering from a head injury sustained in a fall downstairs. He insists that the patient in the next room is his daughter and tries to see her.

   _____

   _____

   _____

3. Mrs. Bell is pacing in the corridor. The nurse said in report that she may be experiencing delirium. She repeatedly asks the same question of the staff. She sometimes bites and spits at others. List factors that cause delirium.

   _____

   _____

   _____

RELATING TO THE NURSING PROCESS

_____

Write the step of the nursing process that is related to the nursing assistant action.

Nursing Assistant Action	Nursing Process Step
1. The nursing assistant listens but does not argue even though the patient's belief is clearly wrong.	_____
2. The nursing assistant reports the patient's use of profanity without labeling his behavior.	_____
3. The nurse observes the way the patient says words and the body language she uses at the time.	_____
4. The nursing assistant reports to the nurse about ways he has found to help the patient deal with stress.	_____
5. The nursing assistant acts in a positive way when a patient is depressed.	_____
6. The nursing assistant reports that the patient is apathetic and having crying spells.	_____
7. The nursing assistant gives instructions slowly and clearly, in simple words, to a disoriented person.	_____

DEVELOPING GREATER INSIGHT

Complete the chart to demonstrate your understanding of the concept of how people cope with stress.

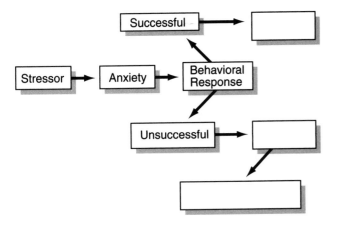

Caring for Patients with Cognitive Impairment and Related Conditions

OBJECTIVES

After completing this unit, you will be able to:

- Spell and define terms.
- Describe the care of persons with mental retardation or developmental disability.
- List eight diseases that may cause dementia, and give an overview of each.
- List the stages of Alzheimer's disease and briefly describe each stage.
- Describe actions to use when working with persons who have dementia.
- Describe the management of patients who wander.

UNIT SUMMARY

- *Cognitive impairment* is a term used to describe deterioration in mental function caused by injury or disease. Persons with cognitive impairment have difficulty learning, processing, and remembering information. They have difficulty planning and carrying out activities of daily living. Short-term memory, intellectual capacity, and safety judgment are impaired.

- Persons with mental retardation (MR) have lower-than-average intelligence, limited ability to learn, and social immaturity. Some can care for themselves and live independently, but those who are severely retarded require lifelong care.

- Developmental disability (DD) first occurs before the age of 22. Persons with this condition have a physical impairment, mental impairment, or a combination of both. Some individuals are born with developmental disability; others acquire the problem before the age of 22 as a result of illness, infection, or trauma.

- Mental decline is not a normal part of aging. However, the risk of mental deterioration increases with age.

- The term *dementia* refers to any disorder of the brain that causes deficits in thinking, memory, and judgment. It is a permanent condition that is not related to acute physical problems.

- Alzheimer's disease is the most common form of dementia. Other types are:

  o Vascular dementia (also called multi-infarct dementia)

  o Huntington's disease

  o Lewy body dementia

  o Parkinson's disease

  o Tertiary syphilis

  o Creutzfeldt-Jakob disease

  o Prion diseases

NURSING ASSISTANT ALERT

Action	Benefit
When caring for patients with cognitive impairment, mental retardation, and developmental disability, ensure a safe environment and teach safety.	Prevents injury.
Be patient, providing information in a slow, simple manner, repeating as needed and using praise liberally.	Reduces frustration and untoward behaviors, promotes positive self-esteem.
Keep instructions simple, avoid rushing, and reduce stress and anxiety.	Prevents agitation, anxiety, and catastrophic reactions.

ACTIVITIES

Vocabulary Exercise

Complete the crossword puzzle by using the definitions in the following clues.

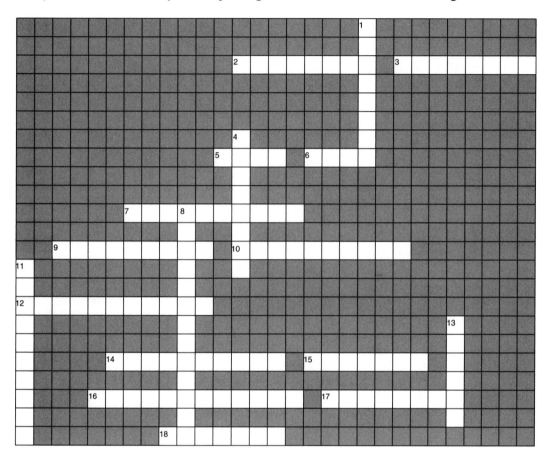

Across

2/3 _____ _____ is
    believed to be caused by a series of strokes.

5/6 _____ _____
    dementia gets its name because of the round
    nerve cell deposits found in the brain after death.

7   Behavior in which a person becomes more
    agitated and disoriented during the evening
    hours.

9/10 Deterioration in mental function caused by injury
    or disease

12 A person with mental _____ has
    lower-than-normal intellectual function.

14/15 _____ _____ is the
    most common cause of dementia.

16/17 A _____ _____ is a
    response to overwhelming stress.

18 Wandering away from the health care facility

Down

1   A person with _____ syphilis
    has neurologic problems and brain damage.

4   A disorder of the brain that causes deficits in
    thinking, memory, and judgment.

8   A _____ disability is present at
    birth or develops before age 22.

8   _____ disease is caused by a
    deficiency of a chemical in brain; persons with
    this condition experience tremors and rigidity.

13 Proteinaceous infectious particles that are
    ingested through infected food, such as meat.

Completion

Complete the following statements by filling in the terms from the list provided.

abnormal behavior	afraid	Alzheimer's disease	bathroom
care plan	communication	consent	dignity
displeasure	distract	harm	masturbation
modify	reason	restraints	rights
safety judgment	stress	sundowning	unmet needs

1. A confused patient may disrobe when she needs to use the _____.

2. Applying _____ may worsen agitation.

3. Nursing assistants may need to _____ their behavior in response to the patient's behavior.

4. Always report _____ to the nurse, even if you believe the behavior is "normal for the patient."

5. When assisting patients with behavior problems, follow the approaches listed on the _____ _____ in the order listed.

6. Maintaining the _____ and self-esteem of patients is important.

7. _____ is an acceptable behavior as long as it is done in a private area.

8. Adults have a legal right to do whatever is pleasing to them, as long as it is not medically contraindicated and both partners are mentally capable of _____.

9. Identifying and modifying the patient's agenda, feelings, and _____ _____ will usually modify or stop wandering behavior.

10. When the ability to use speech is lost, _____ occurs through nonverbal means.

11. _____ _____ is the most common form of dementia.

12. Persons with cognitive impairment have poor _____ _____.

13. Patients with delusions of persecution fear that others will _____ them.

14. _____ means that the patient commonly wanders in the evening and at night.

15. A catastrophic reaction is a response to overwhelming _____.

16. Patients with Alzheimer's disease lose the ability to _____.

17. You may be able to _____ a wandering patient with food or drink.

18. Persons with cognitive impairment have the same legal _____ as everyone else.

19. Biting, scratching, and kicking may be the only way a patient can express _____.

20. Some persons with cognitive impairment are _____ of water.

Short Answer

Briefly answer the following questions in the space provided.

1. List at least 10 guidelines for managing behavior problems.

_____

_____

_____

_____

_____

_____

_____

_____

_____

2. Describe how to manage a patient who makes sexual advances to the nursing assistant.

_____

_____

_____

_____

_____

_____

_____

_____

_____

_____

3. List four reasons for disrobing behavior.

_____

_____

_____

_____

4. List at least 10 guidelines for managing wandering behavior.

_____

_____

_____

_____

_____

_____

_____

_____

_____

_____

True/False

Mark the following true or false by circling T or F.

1.   T   F   Cognitive impairment is a normal aging change.

2.   T   F   In the early stages of Alzheimer's, the person may try to cover for the memory loss.

3.   T   F   Seeing a hat, coat, and keys may trigger wandering.

4.   T   F   Vascular dementia is caused by prions.

5.   T   F   Prions are tiny bacteria found outdoors.

6.   T   F   Persons with Parkinson's disease always develop dementia.

7.   T   F   A person with early-stage Alzheimer's will usually recognize family members.

8.   T   F   Sundowning begins in the third stage of Alzheimer's.

9.   T   F   A patient with cognitive impairment may interpret nursing assistant assistance with peri care
         as a sexual assault.

10.   T   F   Persons with dementia do well in large groups or competitive activities.

11.   T   F   Persons with mental retardation have no capacity for learning.

12.   T   F   Persons with developmental disability are also mentally retarded.

13.   T   F   Developmental disabilities occur before age 18.

14.   T   F   Some individuals with developmental disabilities are independent.

15.   T   F   Quality of life is not a concern in the care of persons with mental retardation and
         developmental disability.

16.   T   F   Persons with mental retardation and developmental disability respond well to praise.

Hidden Picture

Using the following picture, identify the problems that should be corrected (there are 13 total).

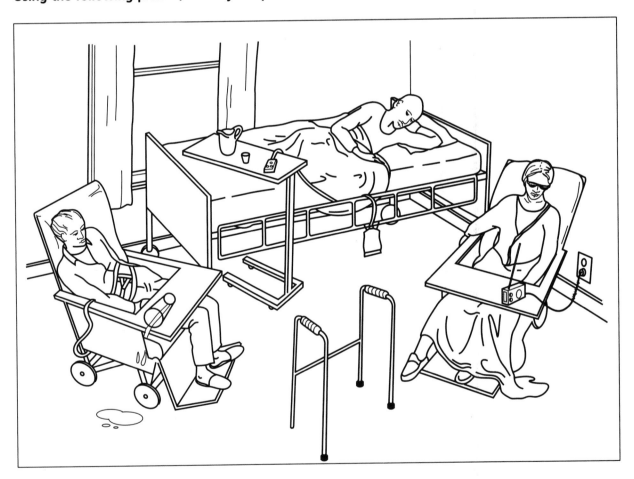

1. _____

2. _____

3. _____

4. _____

5. _____

6. _____

7. _____

8. _____

9. _____

10. _____

11. _____

12. _____

13. _____

RELATING TO THE NURSING PROCESS

Write the step of the nursing process that is related to the nursing assistant action.

Nursing Assistant Action	Nursing Process Step
1. The nursing assistant reassures the patients in his care that they will not be abandoned.	_____
2. The nursing assistant treats each patient with respect.	_____
3. The nursing assistant reports that the patient has complained of feeling sad and lonely.	_____
4. The nursing assistant encourages the cognitively impaired patient to feed himself, but is ready to assist if needed.	_____
5. The nursing assistant encourages the cognitively impaired patient to drink fluids frequently.	_____
6. The nursing assistant checks the wandering patient's whereabouts.	_____
7. The nursing assistant uses gestures to help communicate meaning when the cognitively impaired patient does not understand.	_____

DEVELOPING GREATER INSIGHT

Answer the questions below based on the following situation.

You are working as a nursing assistant on the 3:00 PM to 11:00 PM shift at the Quality Care Convalescent Center. Dr. Zeleski is a 57-year-old patient with Alzheimer's disease. He was formerly a college professor. His hair is "salt-and-pepper" black and gray. He is a well-groomed, good-looking man with a dignified appearance who dresses in color-coordinated sweaters and casual slacks. Dr. Zeleski has good communication skills, and seems to be alert during a brief conversation. When you visit for longer periods of time, you realize that he is very disoriented and does not use good judgment. Because of his good communication skills, age, and appearance, he is often mistaken for a visitor in the facility.

Dr. Zeleski's wife cared for him at home until she had a stroke and was hospitalized. She is in the subacute unit of the local hospital. The patient's daughter tried to care for the doctor in her home, but gave up after several days. The doctor left food unattended on the stove, and forgot the burners were on. He wandered outside in the middle of the night on several occasions. The temperature was very cold and he was not appropriately dressed. Fortunately, his daughter was a very light sleeper. She nailed long chains of loud jingle bells over the doors, so if he went outside, the bells would awaken her. This approach was successful, but having her father in the house was very stressful for the daughter's family.

Because of the patient's lack of safety awareness, they feared he would accidentally burn the house down or wander off and die of exposure or be hit by a car. They admitted him to the Quality Care facility, and made arrangements for his wife to be admitted when she is discharged from the hospital. Dr. Zeleski is currently in a room by himself, in anticipation of his wife's arrival within the next few days. Family members have cautioned the facility that he wandered away from home several times, and stated that they would take legal action if he got outside and was injured. Dr. Zeleski is restless and agitated every evening. His balance is good and he moves quickly. He wears a magnetic wandering bracelet, but has managed to remove it twice. He has left the building and gone outside several times. He usually slips into large groups of visitors who are exiting the building.

Dr. Zeleski often wanders about looking for his wife. He does not remember that she is in the hospital. Sometimes he goes into other patients' rooms and upsets them. He tells you he is going home and argues when reminded that he lives in the facility. He seldom wears a coat or dresses appropriately for the weather. Dr. Zeleski is often so distracted that he does not finish a meal before he gets up to wander again. He has lost weight. He has an order for a regular diet with large portions, with nutritional supplements three times daily and PRN. He especially likes the eggnog-flavor supplement. You know he also likes tuna salad sandwiches and deviled eggs. He has an order for restraints if he becomes unmanageable, but these are to be used only as a last resort.

1. Dr. Zeleski is approaching the door when you see him. He says, "Goodbye. I am going home now." What action will you take to keep the patient safe?

_____

_____

_____

_____

_____

2. You are assigned to care for Dr. Zeleski today. Your unit is short of staff, and Dr. Zeleski is very agitated. A number of visitors have been in the facility, and he has tried to leave several times. Each time staff have retrieved him, but you fear you will be in a patient's room and he will slip out. Should you restrain him to keep him safe? Why or why not? If you elect not to apply restraints, how will you ensure the patient's safety?

_____

_____

_____

_____

_____

3. Dr. Zeleski did not eat his dinner. He got up from the table and started wandering the halls. Almost everyone is in the dining room, and you fear he will go out the door. When you approach the patient, he says he is "late for work." You walk with him as he heads for the door. How can you assist this patient to eat dinner and keep him from leaving the facility?

_____

_____

_____

_____

4. Dr. Zeleski refused to eat his meal. How can you assist in meeting his nutritional needs?

_____

_____

_____

_____

_____

5. Based on the descriptions in your text book, what is Dr. Zeleski's risk for leaving the facility unnoticed? Are there any other factors that increase this patient's chances of eloping successfully? If so, list them.

_____

_____

_____

_____

_____

6. Why are good teamwork and communication important in the care of this patient?

_____

_____

_____

_____

_____

7. You are asked to attend Dr. Zeleski's care conference. The nurse tells you to think about suggestions to keep the patient safe. What will you suggest?

_____

_____

_____

_____

_____

Caring for the Bariatric Patient

After completing this unit, you will be able to:

- Spell and define terms.

- Define the terms *overweight, obesity,* and *morbid obesity,* and explain how these conditions differ from each other.

- Explain why weight affects life span (longevity) and health.

- Define comorbidities and explain how they affect a person's health.

- Describe nursing assistant actions and observations related to the care of patients of size.

- Explain why environmental modifications are needed for bariatric patient care.

- Describe observations to make and methods of meeting bariatric patients' ADL needs.

- List precautions to take when moving and positioning bariatric patients.

UNIT SUMMARY

The incidence of overweight and obesity in the United States is increasing, affecting about one in three adults. The rise in obesity has been rapid in children. As a result, more patients with conditions related to overweight are being admitted to the hospital, and staff must know how to care for them safely and meet their unique needs. Some patients will be admitted for medical problems; others are admitted for bariatric surgery. Comorbidities must be treated and stabilized before surgery can be done. A team effort is essential to good patient care.

- Obesity has many causes, including heredity.

- Body mass index (BMI) is a mathematical calculation used to determine whether a person is at a healthy, normal weight; is overweight; or is obese.

- Obesity is usually considered being overweight by 20% to 30% of the ideal body weight.

- Obesity negatively affects every body system, increases the risk of other serious medical problems, and results in a shorter life span if untreated.

- Persons with obesity experience discrimination and prejudice, difficulty in performing ADLs, and limited access to public facilities. They may also have relationship problems or be victims of physical and psychological abuse. When they are hospitalized, they know that their size makes it hard for staff to care for them, and they may come to your unit with feelings of shame, embarrassment, and fear.

- It is essential to support patients' dignity and self-esteem.

Bariatrics is a relatively new field of medicine that focuses on the treatment and control of obesity and medical conditions and diseases associated with obesity. Environmental modifications and special equipment and supplies are needed in the care of bariatric patients.

Nursing assistants must keep patient and personal safety in mind when caring for bariatric patients. Situations for which the assistant may need special equipment and/or additional help are:

- Moving and positioning the patient

- Assisting with ADLs and toileting

- Mobility and ambulation

The skin is the largest organ of the body; the skin of the bariatric patient usually has been stretched and is easily injured. Provide care to prevent injury from moisture, pressure, friction, and shear force. Bariatric patients are at very high risk of complications when they are immobile.

NURSING ASSISTANT ALERT

Action	Benefit
Attend continuing education classes to learn how to meet the physical and emotional care needs of the bariatric patient.	Expand your nursing assistant knowledge for personal benefit and to meet the needs of a new patient population.
Become familiar with bariatric equipment and how to use it.	Ensures nursing assistant and patient safety.
Monitor for and report potential risk factors, complications, and unsafe situations.	Ensures timely assessment and intervention to improve patient outcomes.
Meet patients' emotional and psychosocial needs through empathy, sensitivity, and compassionate caring.	Promotes patient satisfaction with care and enhances self-esteem.
Monitor for and actively provide nursing care to reduce risk factors and prevent complications of immobility.	Enhances patient confidence and comfort. Helps eliminate complications and comorbidities.

Vocabulary Exercise

Find the following words in the puzzle. *Words in parentheses are not in the puzzle.* **In the space provided, write a definition of each word.**

t	d	B	M	I	L	O	z	r	u	U	I	s	b
a	h	i	Y	I	q	V	A	N	t	F	u	s	a
d	U	g	b	b	B	I	E	H	b	n	e	V	r
v	H	T	i	r	E	J	A	q	n	i	l	x	i
o	H	b	f	e	o	g	l	a	t	O	S	Y	a
c	E	n	h	Y	w	m	p	i	r	R	Q	v	t
a	B	i	v	a	Q	r	d	L	h	S	O	M	r
t	z	c	V	C	m	i	e	I	K	a	l	H	i
e	K	G	e	u	b	s	b	v	I	y	k	T	c
r	Q	n	R	r	n	y	H	Q	o	a	p	v	p
H	d	B	o	Y	C	M	r	A	B	l	e	d	z
X	a	m	S	i	s	W	Q	N	B	h	a	d	l
d	o	o	b	e	s	i	t	y	P	j	P	n	i
c	p	a	n	n	i	c	u	l	u	s	a	Y	k

1. advocate

_____

2. bariatric

_____

3. BMI

_____

4. comorbidities

_____

5. ideal (body weight)

_____

6. morbid (obesity)

_____

7. obesity

_____

8. overweight

_____

9. panniculus

_____

10. pannus

_____

True/False

Mark the following true or false by circling T or F.

1. T   F   A person who is overweight has a BMI of more than 50.

2. T   F   Most obese people eat an enormous amount of food and lack willpower.

3. T   F   Obesity negatively affects every system of the body.

4. T   F   Obesity is commonly hereditary; environmental factors have no effect on weight.

5. T   F   Obesity is a considered a chronic condition.

6. T   F   A fat baby is a healthy baby.

7. T   F   The BMI is the best indicator of an individual's health status.

8. T   F   Comorbidities are diseases and medical conditions that are either caused by or contributed to by morbid obesity.

9. T   F   The weight of an obese person's chest makes breathing more difficult.

10. T   F   The bariatric nurse specialist writes the dietary plan of care and supervises the menu.

11. T   F   The bariatric patient cannot develop malnutrition or dehydration because of the nutrient stores in the adipose tissue.

12. T   F   Bariatric patients often sweat profusely.

13. T   F   Gore-Tex and nylon sheets have a slippery surface that reduces friction and shear and makes it easier to move the patient.

14. T   F   If the patient is too large for the regular scale, obtain the freight scale or laundry scale from the maintenance department.

15. T   F   The patient advocate's main responsibility is protecting the bariatric patient's dignity.

16. T   F   Do not ask the patient what works for his or her care, because it will appear that you do not know what you are doing.

17. T   F   A regular washcloth and towel may be very irritating to the skin of some bariatric patients.

18. T   F   Bariatric patients may need extra fluids to support their body needs.

19. T   F   A condom catheter is commonly used for male bariatric patients because it is easier than inserting a regular catheter, stays in place well, and requires less frequent peri care.

20. T   F   Bariatric patients seldom develop pressure ulcers because of the extra padding over bony prominences.

21. T   F   One staff person should never lift or move more than 55 pounds of body weight without extra help or a mechanical device.

22. T   F   Two or more nursing assistants are often needed to assist the bariatric patient with personal hygiene procedures.

23. T   F   Using the modified Trendelenburg position when moving the bariatric patient up in bed makes the job easier and reduces the risk of injury.

Short Answer

Briefly answer the following questions.

1. When the patient is positioned on his or her side, you should _____

_____

2. Why does the obese patient walk with a wide-based gait? _____

_____

3. The nurse may instruct you to apply an abdominal binder prior to moving the bariatric patient. Why is this done?

_____

_____

4. If a standing bariatric patient begins to fall to the floor, what is the most important action to take?

_____

_____

_____

RELATING TO THE NURSING PROCESS

Write the step of the nursing process that is related to the nursing assistant action.

Nursing Assistant Action	Nursing Process Step
1. The nursing assistant finds that the patient's blood pressure is 180/106, so she rechecks it. Finding the value the same, she seeks out the nurse to report her findings.	_____
2. The nurse has given Mr. Mulvaney an insulin injection. He instructs the nursing assistant to monitor for signs of hypoglycemia, to recheck the blood sugar in 2 hours, and to report the value.	_____
3. Mr. Mulvaney's plan of care is not working and the patient is dissatisfied. The nurse asks the nursing assistant about care plan approaches that have been effective, and which approaches have not worked.	_____
4. The nursing assistant notifies the nurse that Ms. Turpel, a recent bariatric surgery patient, is vomiting.	_____
5. The nursing assistant gets another assistant to help her perform peri care on Mrs. Evert.	_____

Caring for the Patient Who Is Dying

OBJECTIVES

After completing this unit, you will be able to:

- Spell and define terms.
- Describe the grieving process and list the steps.
- Describe the nursing assistant's responsibilities for providing supportive care.
- Describe the hospice philosophy and method of care.
- List the signs of approaching death.
- Demonstrate Procedure 85 (set out in this unit in the textbook).

UNIT SUMMARY

Assisting with terminal and postmortem care is a difficult but essential part of nursing assistant duties. It requires a high degree of sensitivity, understanding, and tact.

- Both the patient and the family require support during this trying period.

- The religious preferences and cultural practices of the patient and the family must be respected and provided for.

- The procedure for postmortem care must be carried out with efficiency and respect.

NURSING ASSISTANT ALERT

Action	Benefit
Recognize that the stages of grief are experienced by both patient and family.	Allows staff to provide essential emotional support.
Remember that people react to a terminal diagnosis in a variety of ways.	Permits nursing care to be individualized.
Identify the signs of impending death.	Allows proper nursing care interventions to be carried out.
Treat the body with the same respect as a living patient.	Maintains dignity and respect.
Apply the principles of standard precautions after death.	Prevents the spread of infection.

ACTIVITIES

Vocabulary Exercise

Each line has four different spellings of a word. Circle the correctly spelled word.

1. critical   cretical   critecal   creticale
2. posmortum   postmartem   postmortem   postmortom
3. hopice   hopise   hospise   hospice
4. terminale   terminal   termanel   termanal
5. danial   deniel   denial   deniale
6. morabund   moribund   moreband   moribond
7. annointing   anointing   annointen   anontin
8. awtopsie   awtopsy   autopse   autopsy
9. bargaining   bargenan   bargainin   bergaining
10. rigor mortis rigor mortus   riger mortis   regor mortos

Completion

Complete the statements in the spaces provided.

1. When the patient's condition is critical, the _____ places the patient's name on the critical list.

2. Sacrament of the Sick is requested for the patient of the _____ faith.

3. Hospice care is based on the philosophy that death is a _____ process.

4. Hospice care is provided for people with a life expectancy of _____.

5. Hospice care is provided by _____ who work with the patient and the family.

6. As death approaches, body functions _____.

7. The last sense lost is the sense of _____.

8. As death approaches, the pulse becomes _____ and progressively _____.

9. The time of death is determined by the _____ .

10. Under no circumstances should the _____ inform the family of the patient's death.

11. As a nursing assistant, you have a unique opportunity to be a source of _____ and _____ to the dying patient and the family.

12. During the time the patient is dying, you must provide the family and patient with _____.

13. The nursing assistant must realize that dying is a _____ each person must make _____.

True/False

Mark the following true or false by circling T or F.

1. T F A patient goes through each stage of grieving in a sequential order.

2. T F Once he or she has moved on to another stage of the grieving process, the patient never returns to the former stage.

3. T F All patients go through each stage of grieving at the same rate.

4. T F The nursing assistant must have an understanding attitude during each stage of the grieving process.

5. T F The family members may go through the same five stages of grief.

6. T F The nursing assistant should reflect the patient's statements during the stage of denial.

7. T F If the patient seems depressed, it is best to leave him alone to work it out himself.

8. T F The patient in the stage of acceptance has no fear.

9. T F The stage of depression is often filled with expression of regrets.

10. T F The patient who has reached the stage of acceptance may try to assist those around her to deal with her death.

11. T F The durable power of attorney rule goes into effect as soon as a patient is admitted to a health care facility.

12. T F Supportive care for terminally ill patients does not include life-sustaining treatments.

Short Answer

Briefly answer the following questions in the spaces provided.

1. Write the five stages of grief as outlined by E. Kübler-Ross.

   a. _____

   b. _____

   c. _____

   d. _____

   e. _____

2. What are the goals of hospice programs?

   a. _____

   b. _____

   c. _____

3. As a member of the hospice team, how can you promote the hospice philosophy?

   a. _____

   b. _____

   c. _____

   d. _____

4. What are five moribund changes?

   a. _____

   b. _____

   c. _____

   d. _____

   e. _____

5. What items would you expect to find in a morgue kit?

   a. _____

   b. _____

   c. _____

   d. _____

   e. _____

6. What should you do before moving the body to the morgue, to prevent upsetting other patients?

   _____

   _____

7. Why is the use of standard precautions necessary when performing postmortem care?

   _____

   _____

Clinical Situations

Briefly describe how a nursing assistant should react to the following situations.

1. Your terminal patient, who had been crying earlier, suddenly appears cheerful and talks about a trip he is planning for next year.

   _____

   _____

2. The patient expresses a desire to see her clergyperson.

   _____

   _____

3. The physician has pronounced the patient deceased and you are to prepare the patient for the return of the family.

   a. _____

   b. _____

   c. _____

   d. _____

   e. _____

4. The patient has an order for supportive care only. Explain what care this includes.

   a. _____

   b. _____

   c. _____

   d. _____

5. The patient has both a living will and a durable power of attorney. Write the name of the document that assigns responsibility for making health care decisions for the patient.

   _____

6. A patient has a no-code order. State how this order influences care if the patient experiences respiratory and cardiac arrest.

   _____

RELATING TO THE NURSING PROCESS

Write the step of the nursing process that is related to the nursing assistant action.

Nursing Assistant Action	Nursing Process Step
1. The nursing assistant promptly reports a terminally ill patient's complaints of pain to the nurse.	_____
2. During the postmortem period, the nursing assistant cares for the body with dignity.	_____
3. The nursing assistant checks the dying patient frequently and keeps the nurse informed of changes in condition.	_____
4. The nursing assistant offers quiet support to the family of the dying patient by listening.	_____

DEVELOPING GREATER INSIGHT

Answer the questions below based upon the following situation.

Mrs. Kosmacek has a terminal diagnosis, and her condition has been steadily declining. She keeps talking about a trip she plans to take next summer, which is 10 months away. She has been planning this trip and saving her money for many years. She says she is going to Poland to research her ancestry. While she is overseas, she plans to go on to the Vatican to see if she can get a blessing from the pope. She says she is going to make reservations soon and make a large, nonrefundable deposit so she gets the dates and accommodations she wants.

1. How will you react to the patient's discussion of trip plans?

   _____

   _____

   _____

   _____

2. Will you report this conversation to anyone? If so, to whom and why?

_____

_____

_____

_____

3. What stage of the grieving process is the patient displaying?

_____

_____

_____

_____

Fill in the chart to identify the stages of the grieving process and nursing assistant response.

Patient Statement	Stage of Grief	Nursing Assistant Response
4. "I should donate to the cancer charity so they find a cure in time."		
5. "They haven't visited in two days. No one cares about me any more."		
6. "I need to speak with my cousin, Charles. We haven't spoken in years, and it's time."		
7. "This diagnosis can't be right. The doctor doesn't know what she's doing."		
8. "This food makes me sick. In fact, I'm sick of all of you. Take this horrible food out of here."		

Other Health Care Settings

The Nursing Assistant in Home Care

OBJECTIVES

After completing this unit, you will be able to:

- Spell and define terms.
- Describe the characteristics that are important in the nursing assistant who provides home care.
- List at least 10 methods of protecting your personal safety when working as a home care assistant in the community.
- Describe the duties of the nursing assistant who works in the home setting.
- Describe the duties of the homemaker assistant.
- Carry out home care activities needed to maintain a safe and clean environment.

UNIT SUMMARY

There is an increasing trend to provide home health care to housebound, recuperating, and chronically ill clients. The nursing assistant who provides this care may also carry out housekeeping activities.

Home health care consists of:

- Maintaining a safe, comfortable environment for the client
- Managing infection control
- Carrying out proper nursing techniques under the supervision of the nurse care coordinator

The home health assistant occupies the position of a:

- Member of the home health care team
- Guest in the client's home
- Provider of direct health care and household assistance

NURSING ASSISTANT ALERT

Action	Benefit
Adapt procedures to the home setting following accepted techniques and safety standards.	Ensures that the same standard of care is given in all health care settings.
Carry out housekeeping duties diligently.	Secures a clean and safe environment for the client.
Be alert to unsafe conditions in the home, and correct or report them.	Prevents injury to client and caregiver.
Adapt procedures to equipment found in the home whenever possible.	Contributes to cost containment.

ACTIVITIES

Vocabulary Exercise

y	i	r	t	n	a	t	s	i	s	s	a	l
i	t	n	r	e	i	r	r	a	b	m	e	e
n	o	e	t	g	r	c	z	j	a	v	s	i
f	r	j	f	e	a	g	f	e	a	r	h	s
e	g	u	b	a	r	b	t	r	u	n	t	e
c	a	z	x	u	s	m	t	n	c	a	t	i
t	n	i	a	l	m	~	i	t	y	q	m	l
i	i	r	l	a	e	t	h	t	o	t	d	p
o	z	b	p	m	n	d	z	e	t	q	p	p
u	e	a	i	e	d	d	x	q	e	e	l	u
s	q	t	i	c	j	z	s	w	v	d	n	s
q	k	l	a	l	c	o	h	o	l	m	i	t
s	c	h	o	m	e	m	a	k	e	r	j	a

1. Find these words in the puzzle and circle them:

aide	alcohol	assistant
bag	barrier	client
homemaker	infectious	intermittent
map	nurse	organize
safety	supplies	team
time/travel		

Completion

Complete the following statements in the spaces provided.

1. The nursing assistant contributes to the planning step of the nursing process by actively participating in _____.

2. The client should, if able, make decisions about food _____.

3. The client's bathroom should be cleaned _____.

4. Before _____ the client's appliances, seek _____ from a family member.

5. Be sure to _____ the _____ off before hanging laundered clothes outside.

6. Before storing clothes that have been laundered, check for needed _____.

7. Drip-dry fabrics should be washed _____ so they can be hung and folded.

8. The primary role of the home health assistant is to _____.

9. The major responsibility of the homemaker assistant is to provide _____.

10. In some cases, the nursing assistant who provides health care may be asked to carry out _____ chores.

11. Because home health assistants handle money, they must be _____ people.

12. The home health care assistant's activities are planned around the _____.

13. To save costs, _____ enema equipment may be substituted for disposable enema equipment.

14. Statements of the client that reflect neglect or abuse should be _____.

15. Chemicals such as household cleaning supplies and insecticides should be kept locked up when the client is _____.

16. Dust, dirty dishes, and improper care of foods contribute to the spread of _____.

Short Answer

Briefly answer the following questions in the spaces provided.

1. What are three areas to report that support the assessment process?

    a. _____

    b. _____

    c. _____

2. What are two ways to support the implementation portion of the nursing process?

    a. _____

    b. _____

3. What are two ways to promote the evaluation part of the nursing process?

    a. _____

    b. _____

4. What are three household duties the nursing assistant frequently performs?

    a. _____

    b. _____

    c. _____

5. What are three household cleaning duties not included in the nursing assistant's responsibilities?

   a. _____

   b. _____

   c. _____

6. What are four numbers to be kept close to the telephone during home care?

   a. _____

   b. _____

   c. _____

   d. _____

7. What action should the nursing assistant take when cleaning laundry soiled by blood?

   _____

8. What are 10 ways of maintaining your personal safety when working in home care?

   a. _____

   b. _____

   c. _____

   d. _____

   e. _____

   f. _____

   g. _____

   h. _____

   i. _____

   j. _____

True/False

Mark the following true or false by circling T or F.

1. T   F   Household duties may be part of the home nursing assistant's responsibilities.

2. T   F   Caring for food properly is part of your responsibility.

3. T   F   It is all right to leave dirty dishes in the sink after the client eats.

4. T   F   Cleaning the client's bathroom and kitchen are part of the nursing assistant's responsibilities.

5. T   F   Fresh fruits that are to be used right away should be stored in the refrigerator.

6. T   F   Dried and canned foods should be stored in the refrigerator.

7. T   F   It is proper to leave dairy products unrefrigerated until use.

8. T   F   Frozen foods may safely be thawed in the kitchen sink until use.

9. T   F   Dirty dishes left to accumulate will contribute to infection.

10. T   F   Loose scatter rugs are safe to use in the home if the client knows where they are placed.

11. T   F   Electrical outlets that have multiple cords plugged in could cause fires.

Clinical Situations

Briefly describe what the nursing assistant could do to meet the following needs in the home setting.

1. The bed is not flexible and the client needs to be in a semi-Fowler's position.

   _____

2. The client has sprained an ankle and there is no ice bag to apply cold.

   _____

3. The client needs to remain in bed and likes to do puzzles to pass the time.

   _____

4. The client is very heavy and there is no trapeze to help with lifting and moving.

   _____

5. You must give a bed bath and there is no bath blanket.

   _____

6. The client must remain in bed, so all care must be given on a regular-height twin bed.

   _____

7. The client is a child who, though in traction, has many toys, crayons, and books scattered over the bed.

   _____

8. You need a place to put soiled laundry as you give care.

   _____

9. The client occasionally needs an enema, and disposable enema equipment is too expensive.

   _____

10. The client has an upper respiratory infection, and you must safely dispose of soiled tissues.

    _____

11. You are visiting Mrs. Morrison regularly as part of your assignment. This morning you notice a bruise on her arm and she tells you that she and her daughter, who lives with her, quarreled last evening. What action should you take?

    _____

    _____

12. Mary Schroeder is 91 years of age and is very frail. She has been diagnosed with emphysema, CHF, and diabetes. She is being cared for by her sister, who is 93 years old. You are assigned to provide personal hygiene care three mornings each week. Ms. Schroeder is in a regular bed that is low to the floor and cannot have its position changed. The client is incontinent. You must adapt her low-income environment to provide proper care.

    _____

    _____

    _____

RELATING TO THE NURSING PROCESS

Write the step of the nursing process that is related to the nursing assistant action.

Nursing Assistant Action   **Nursing Process Step**

1. The nursing assistant reports to her supervisor improvement in the homebound client's appetite.   _____

2. The nursing assistant reports that the client receiving home care is now able to function independently.   _____

3. The nursing assistant informs the supervisor that stress between the client and his daughter about the client's planned activities is interfering with the client's recovery.   _____

DEVELOPING GREATER INSIGHT

Answer the questions below based upon the following situation.

Mr. Hillhouse has terminal cancer. You will spend an entire shift with him. You must give him a bed bath, change his linen, and prepare his meals. The client enjoys playing cards and dominoes. Your odometer reads 53726 when you leave your home, and 53735 when you arrive at the client's home. Your time in is 7:00 AM. You leave the client's home at 3:40 PM. Your odometer reads 53735 when you leave the client's home and 53744 when you arrive at your own home.

1. Compute the total time spent with the client.

_____

_____

_____

2. Compute the total mileage.

_____

_____

_____

3. Your work is done by 1:00 PM and the client is watching television. He says he does not want to take a nap. Mr. Hillhouse says he is bored with the soap operas. Describe your actions.

_____

_____

_____

_____

Body Systems, Common Disorders, and Related Care Procedures

UNIT **35**

Caring for Patients with Disorders of the Integumentary System

OBJECTIVES

After completing this unit, you will be able to:

- Spell and define terms.

- Review the location and function of the skin.

- Identify aging changes of the integumentary system.

- List common problems related to the integumentary system.

- Identify observations of signs and symptoms that the nursing assistant should make and report.

- Identify patients at risk for the formation of pressure ulcers.

- Describe the stages of pressure ulcer formation.

- Describe measures and identify appropriate nursing assistant actions to prevent pressure ulcers.

- Describe electrical, thermal, and chemical burns.

- Demonstrate Procedure 86 (set out in this unit in the textbook).

UNIT SUMMARY

- The skin is the largest organ of the human body. The condition of the skin indicates the general health of the body. The skin protects against infection, maintains fluid balance, excretes waste products, maintains temperature, and provides sensation for the body.

- Aging changes cause the skin to become very dry and fragile. The skin of elderly persons often tears, breaks, and bruises readily. Handle elderly patients very gently.

- Observation of the skin and accurate descriptions of what you see must be carefully charted. Abnormalities should be reported to the nurse.

- Pressure ulcers result from pressure on one area of the body that interferes with circulation. Pressure ulcers:

  o Are more easily prevented than cured

  o May occur in any patient

  o Occur in stages that are recognizable and treatable

- The five most common conditions in which pressure ulcers develop are pneumonia, urinary tract infection, septicemia, aspiration pneumonitis, and congestive heart failure.

- Burns:

  o Are classified according to the depth of tissue damage

  o Require special care, often in burn centers

- Your bandage scissors, stethoscope, and other personal items may transfer pathogens from one patient to the next. If personal equipment items will be used during a procedure, wash them with an alcohol product or soap and water before and after each use. If you use a cloth stethoscope tubing cover, wash it each day with your uniform. Carry extra covers so you can change the cover if it becomes contaminated.

NURSING ASSISTANT ALERT

Action	Benefit
Observe and carefully describe and report skin lesions.	Establishes proper data for more accurate evaluation.
Identify patients at risk for pressure ulcers.	Allows timely nursing interventions.
Carry out pressure ulcer care as prescribed.	Limits more extensive damage. Promotes repair.

ACTIVITIES

Vocabulary Exercise

Complete the word search puzzle by finding and circling the words in the following list. Define the words on the lines below.

n	s	z	f	n	o	i	t	c	i	r	f	e
d	o	n	l	e	s	i	o	n	s	e	s	s
n	s	i	r	p	k	s	m	b	c	c	d	k
a	i	b	t	u	w	b	n	c	h	s	e	i
m	s	b	z	a	b	u	h	a	m	m	m	n
o	o	x	o	b	i	y	r	y	s	y	n	-
t	r	r	m	q	m	r	d	l	p	g	o	t
a	c	m	n	o	r	y	o	c	u	u	i	e
m	e	y	s	a	t	c	s	c	x	i	s	a
e	n	i	s	a	z	m	c	y	x	n	a	r
h	s	h	v	m	e	e	p	v	u	e	r	u
l	a	c	e	r	a	t	i	o	n	m	b	y
c	o	n	t	u	s	i	o	n	d	h	a	u

1. abrasion

_____

2. ecchymosis

_____

3. contusion

_____

4. hematoma

_____

5. friction

_____

6. rash

_____

7. lesions

_____

8. eschar

_____

9. necrosis

_____

10. excoriation

_____

11. laceration

_____

12. skin-tear

_____

13. burns

_____

Anatomy Review

Identify the stage of each pressure ulcer. Identify the primary areas of affected tissue in the spaces provided.

1.

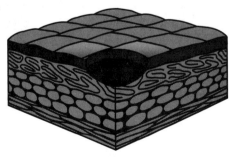

_____

_____

2.

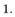
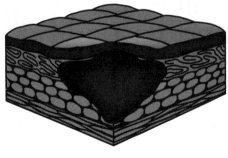

_____

_____

3.

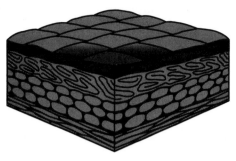

_____

_____

_____

4.

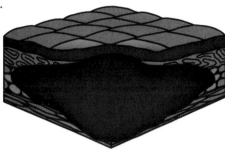

_____

_____

_____

Completion

Complete the following statements in the spaces provided.

1. Clean dressings are used on _____ and _____ wounds.

2. Wrap a bandage from _____ to _____ .

3. Check the circulation _____ to a bandage to ensure that the blood flow is not occluded.

4. Patients with skin lesions must be handled _____ without _____ the skin.

5. Pressure ulcers are more easily _____ than _____ .

6. Obese patients have a/an _____ risk of pressure ulcers compared with persons of normal size.

7. Reddened skin is a sign of the _____ stage of tissue breakdown.

8. If the epidermis is broken, it should be kept _____ .

9. Indication of infection in a pressure ulcer might include _____ and a foul _____ .

10. A pressure ulcer that looks like a minor blister is a Stage _____ ulcer.

11. In stage 2 breakdown, it is imperative that the _____ be relieved, or more serious damage will occur.

12. Patients who have pressure ulcers are always at high risk of developing _____ .

13. In a stage _____ pressure ulcer, the redness or discoloration does not go away within 30 minutes after pressure has been relieved.

14. Skin lesions may be caused by _____, _____, or _____.

15. _____ your bandage scissors and dry them well _____ and _____ using them during a dressing change.

16. Shearing occurs when skin moves in one direction while structures underneath _____.

17. Patients with stage 4 pressure ulcers experience _____ and _____ and are at great risk for infection.

18. Various _____ may be used to relieve pressure, friction, and shearing on specific areas of the body.

19. _____ the heels from the surface of the bed to relieve pressure.

20. Patients with _____ fractures are at high risk of developing heel ulcers.

21. Patients using low air loss beds must be _____ every _____ or they will develop pressure ulcers.

22. In a dark-skinned person, a stage 1 pressure ulcer will appear _____ or _____ in color.

23. _____ are injuries that result from scraping the skin.

24. _____ are mechanical injuries (usually caused by a blow) resulting in hemorrhage beneath the unbroken skin.

25. A bruise is also called an _____.

26. A _____ is a localized mass of blood that is confined to one area.

27. _____ are accidental breaks in the skin.

28. Dark purple bruises on the forearms and back of hands that commonly occur in elderly individuals are called _____.

29. _____ are shallow injuries in which the epidermis is torn.

30. Body lice, or _____, are parasites that feed on humans.

31. _____ are mites that cause itching and a rash-like appearance.

32. When applying a clean dressing, handle the dressing only by the _____.

Short Answer

Briefly answer the following questions.

1. How could you best document the following skin lesions?

   a. skin appears scratched or scraped away _____

   b. brown areas of skin that look like large freckles

   _____

   c. dark purple bruises on backs of hands of an elderly person

   _____

2. Which four types of patients are prone to tissue breakdown?

    a. _____

    b. _____

    c. _____

    d. _____

3. What are 12 ways to avoid the development of pressure ulcers?

    a. _____

    b. _____

    c. _____

    d. _____

    e. _____

    f. _____

    g. _____

    h. _____

    i. _____

    j. _____

    k. _____

    l. _____

4. List five nursing assistant measures for care of a patient with burns.

    a. _____

    b. _____

    c. _____

    d. _____

    e. _____

5. List two actions the nursing assistant can take to increase circulation to tissues.

    a. _____

    b. _____

6. Why is it important to prevent skin tears?

    a. _____

    b. _____

    c. _____

7. Mr. French is in fair physical condition. He is rather lethargic and is ambulatory with assistance. He has limited movement of his left arm and leg, is continent, and eats poorly. He has an open lesion over his left hip. He has a scar on his coccyx from a healed pressure ulcer. What is his risk of pressure ulcer development?

_____

8. Complete the turning wheel to demonstrate your understanding of the principle of relieving pressure.

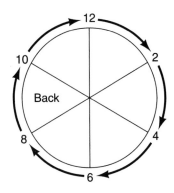

9. List the areas most subject to breakdown when the patient is in the position shown.

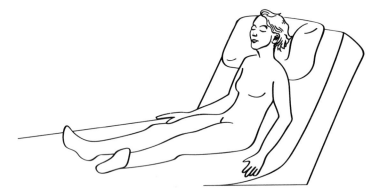

a. _____

b. _____

c. _____

d. _____

e. _____

Clinical Situations

Briefly describe how a nursing assistant should react to the following situations.

1. You burned your finger.

_____

2. You are assigned to give a bed bath and find that the patient has skin lesions.

_____

_____

RELATING TO THE NURSING PROCESS

Write the step of the nursing process that is related to the nursing assistant action.

Nursing Assistant Action   **Nursing Process Step**

1. The nursing assistant charts the presence of excoriation on the
   patient's buttocks.   _____

2. The nursing assistant gently massages the skin, avoiding a reddened area,
   following the nurse's orders.   _____

3. The nursing assistant reports a pustule noted on the patient's thigh.   _____

4. The nursing assistant makes sure the patient's position is changed at least
   every 2 hours.   _____

5. The nursing assistant uses a turning sheet to move dependent patients
   in bed.   _____

6. The nursing assistant reports an area of irritation around the entrance of the
   nasogastric tube into the patient's nose.   _____

7. The nursing assistant informs the nurse that a patient's rash has improved
   since beginning the new treatment.   _____

DEVELOPING GREATER INSIGHT

1. What do the following patients have in common: a patient with a nasogastric tube, a patient with an
   indwelling catheter, and a patient who is able to move independently?

   _____

   _____

   _____

   _____

2. Explain why changes in the aging integumentary system make the elderly more prone to develop
   pressure ulcers.

   _____

   _____

   _____

   _____

Caring for Patients with Cardiopulmonary Disorders

OBJECTIVES

After completing this unit, you will be able to:

- Spell and define terms.
- Identify aging changes of the circulatory and respiratory systems.
- Describe some common disorders of the circulatory and respiratory systems.
- Describe nursing assistant observations and actions related to care of patients with disorders of the circulatory and respiratory systems.
- Identify patients who are at high risk of poor oxygenation.
- Describe nursing assistant care of a patient who is on a ventilator.
- Demonstrate Procedures 87–89 (set out in this unit in the textbook).

UNIT SUMMARY

The cardiovascular system is the transportation system of the body.

- The heart and blood vessels make up a closed network. This network carries the blood and the products of and for metabolism.
- Diseases that affect the heart or blood vessels often have a related effect on many other parts of the body, especially the respiratory tract.
- The organs of respiration function to take in and exchange oxygen and output carbon dioxide. Diseases that affect the respiratory tract make breathing difficult.
- Cardiac and respiratory problems affect patients at the lowest, most basic level of

Maslow's hierarchy of needs, making attention to these problems very important.

- Because heart and pulmonary diseases are so prevalent, the nursing assistant will likely provide care for many patients with cardiopulmonary problems.
- Patients with many cardiopulmonary conditions are at high risk of developing hypoxemia, a serious complication.
- Immobility is a barrier to positive outcomes.
- Capillary refill checks and the pulse oximeter are excellent tools for monitoring patients who are at risk of hypoxemia.

NURSING ASSISTANT ALERT

Action	Benefit
Do nothing to limit circulation.	Allows patient to make optimum use of cardiovascular function.
Recognize that abnormalities in any part of the cardiovascular system may affect other parts of the body and/or the body as a whole.	Alerts staff to the significance of signs and symptoms in other systems.
Carefully observe, report, and document observations.	Provides a database for appropriate nursing interventions.
Use standard precautions when working with patients who have respiratory tract conditions.	Prevents transmission of disease.
Note, report, and document alteration in respiratory patterns or function.	Early interventions can improve ventilation and gas exchange.
Be prepared to react quickly and correctly to prevent emergencies involving oxygen use.	Averts possible fire hazards and patient injury.
Follow procedures for sputum specimen collection carefully.	Avoids contamination of specimens. Protects against transmission of infectious materials.

ACTIVITIES

Vocabulary Exercise

Unscramble the words introduced in this unit and define them.

1. N A Y P E D S _____

_____

2. C G Y Y R T E L A M O N _____

_____

3. L T E P I I S H B _____

_____

4. C E S H I I M A _____

_____

5. E A T T M R C O O S H Y _____

_____

6. P R Y T O H Y E P R H _____

_____

7. I N G N A A _____

_____

8. T C E A S I S _____

_____

9. Y I M X A E O H P _____

_____

10. Y R I D S S A A S C _____

_____

Completion

Complete the following statements in the spaces provided.

1. Patients who have long-standing cardiac disease often develop diseases of the _____ system.

2. Blood vessels that serve the outer parts of the body are called _____ blood vessels.

3. Blood abnormalities are referred to as blood _____.

4. It takes longer for the heart rate to return to normal after _____.

5. _____ develops when the heart cannot pump blood efficiently.

6. Protect the patient's feet from _____.

7. _____ is the most common form of vascular disease, in which lipids are deposited on the walls of arteries.

8. When the coronary muscles are blocked, the heart tissue becomes _____.

9. _____ form when the valves in the veins in the legs become weakened.

10. A patient with _____ has great difficulty breathing if not sitting upright.

11. Symptoms of a URI include runny nose, watery eyes, and _____.

12. It is important for the nursing assistant to know and read the _____ rate of oxygen for each patient.

13. Chronic _____ is prolonged inflammation in the bronchi due to infection or irritants.

14. When a person has _____, the air sacs enlarge and lose their elasticity and ability to recoil.

15. Being unable to _____ is very frightening.

16. Avoid getting _____, _____, _____, or _____ near or in the respiratory stoma.

17. Room air is approximately _____ oxygen.

Short Answer

Briefly answer the following questions.

1. List 10 important things you will do in the care of patients who are mechanically ventilated.

   a. _____

   b. _____

   c. _____

   d. _____

   e. _____

   f. _____

   g. _____

   h. _____

   i. _____

   j. _____

2. List 10 nursing assistant responsibilities in caring for the feet of patients who have peripheral vascular disease.

   a. _____

   b. _____

   c. _____

   d. _____

   e. _____

   f. _____

   g. _____

   h. _____

   i. _____

   j. _____

3. List 10 observations that you would report about a patient with a circulatory disorder.

   a. _____

   b. _____

   c. _____

   d. _____

   e. _____

   f. _____

   g. _____

   h. _____

   i. _____

   j. _____

Hidden Picture

Carefully study the following picture and identify the rules of oxygen safety that have been violated. Write them in the spaces provided. (There are 11.)

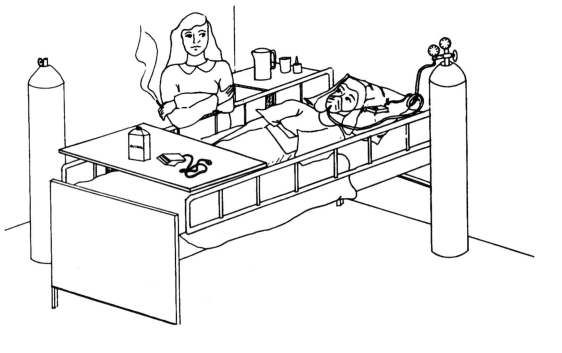

1. _____
2. _____
3. _____
4. _____
5. _____
6. _____
7. _____
8. _____
9. _____
10. _____
11. _____

Clinical Situations

Briefly describe how a nursing assistant should react to the following situations.

1. Your patient, who has angina pectoris, is having an argument with a visitor.

   _____

   _____

2. You are passing out meal trays and find a salt packet on the tray of a patient who has congestive heart failure and is on a sodium-restricted diet.

   _____

3. The patient with congestive heart failure has an erratic radial pulse rate of 72.

   _____

4. You are assigned to collect a sputum specimen for culture and sensitivity. Before collecting a specimen, the patient should

   _____

   _____

5. Complete the following label, which is attached to a specimen container, using the following information: Mr. James Brown is a patient in room 604. His hospital number is 689473. Dr. Smith has ordered a sputum specimen to be taken today for culture.

   Name _____   Room _____

   Date _____   Hospital Number _____

   Doctor _____

   Specimen _____   Examination _____

RELATING TO THE NURSING PROCESS

Write the step of the nursing process that is related to the nursing assistant action.

Nursing Assistant Action	Nursing Process Step
1. The nursing assistant reports that the patient's legs are pale and cool to the touch.	_____
2. The nursing assistant weighs the patient who has congestive heart failure daily.	_____
3. The nursing assistant completes the bath for the patient who has congestive heart failure, to lessen fatigue.	_____
4. The nursing assistant provides special mouth care for the patient who has anemia.	_____
5. The nursing assistant reports that the patient who is anemic tires very easily.	_____
6. The nursing assistant makes sure that the strap holding a nasal cannula delivering oxygen is not too tight.	_____
7. The nursing assistant periodically removes an oxygen delivery mask and washes and dries carefully underneath it.	_____
8. The nursing assistant reports that the patient's respirations have become labored.	_____
9. The nursing assistant keeps the patient's face free of any nasal discharge when a nasal catheter is in use.	_____
10. The nursing assistant positions pillows behind the patient's back to assist his breathing.	_____
11. The nursing assistant helps position the patient so the respiratory therapist can give a treatment.	_____
12. The nursing assistant informs the nurse that the oxygen flow meter is set lower than the level noted on the care plan.	_____

Caring for Patients with Disorders of the Musculoskeletal and Nervous Systems

OBJECTIVES

After completing this unit, you will be able to:

- Spell and define terms.

- Identify aging changes of the musculoskeletal system and nervous system.

- Describe some common conditions of the musculoskeletal system and nervous system.

- Describe nursing assistant actions and observations related to the care of patients with conditions and diseases of the musculoskeletal system and nervous system.

- Demonstrate Procedures 90–91 (set out in this unit in the textbook).

UNIT SUMMARY

- Orthopedic injuries often require long periods of immobilization and rehabilitation.

- Routine range-of-motion exercises must be carried out for all uninjured joints to:

  o Prevent deformities and joint stiffening

  o Promote general circulation

  o Prevent mineral loss from the bones

- Special nursing care for patients with fractures, hip prostheses, joint replacement, and other orthopedic surgery:

  o Ensures proper alignment

  o Prevents pressure areas

  o Avoids skin breakdown

- Continuous passive motion (CPM) therapy is often ordered to reduce the risk of complications following joint replacement and other orthopedic procedures.

- Compartment syndrome is a serious complication of injury and orthopedic surgery. This painful condition occurs when pressure within the muscles builds up, preventing blood and oxygen from reaching muscles and nerves.

- Osteoporosis is a metabolic disorder in which bone mass is lost, causing bones to become porous and spongy and fracture more easily.

- Fibromyalgia is a common chronic pain syndrome for which there is no known cause or cure.

The nursing assistant assists the professional nurse in the care of patients with neurological conditions. Although the nurse is responsible for neurological assessment and intervention, an alert nursing assistant can make valuable observations.

- If the nursing assistants notes changes in level of consciousness, response, or behavior, he reports the changes accurately and promptly.

- Under supervision, the nursing assistant provides specific care for patients who have neurologic disorders related to medical problems and injuries.

Diseases and injuries of the nervous system often require a long recovery period. During the period of convalescence, the nursing assistant plays an important role. Lots of patience, empathy, and skill are needed to assist these patients in their recovery.

NURSING ASSISTANT ALERT

Action	Benefit
Encourage activity that is consistent with individual patient limitations.	Prevents loss of mobility. Helps prevent the development of contractures.
Maintain and promote proper alignment.	Encourages optimum functional ability.
Carry out range-of-motion exercises for patients who are unable to do so themselves.	Maintains mobility and prevents contractures.
Document observations and care accurately.	Provides a database for correct nursing evaluations and interventions.
Patiently use a variety of communication skills.	Lessens patient frustration. Improves accuracy in sending and receiving messages.
Be consistent in care and use established routines.	Requires fewer stressful adjustments for the patient.

ACTIVITIES

Vocabulary Exercise

Each line has four different spellings of a word. Circle the correctly spelled word.

1. athroplasti	arthroplasty	aerthroplesty	arthrouplasty
2. eckymosus	ecckymoses	ecchymosis	eckimoses
3. amputashun	ampetation	amputacion	amputation
4. suppinachon	suppination	supination	suppinasion
5. spika	spyca	spiecka	spica
6. extension	extinsion	extenchon	extention
7. aduction	adducsion	adduchon	adduction
8. dorsiflexion	dorseflexion	dorsiflextion	dorsyflection
9. eavershun	everscion	evirtion	eversion
10. hemiplegia	hemmyplesha	hemyplesia	hemipligia
11. nyestagmis	niestagmus	nystagmus	nistagmis
12. Lermitty's	Lhermitte's	Lermyttie's	Llearmitys
13. tetriplegia	tetraplegia	tetrepleghia	teatriplesha
14. sclerosis	sclairosis	sclearocis	scleroses
15. orra	aura	oera	aerruh

Matching

Match the term on the right with the information on the left. Answers may be used more than once.

1. Repair done for hip fracture	a. cerebrovascular accident
2. Involves only part of the cross-section of bone	b. chorea
3. Loss of ability to express or understand speech	c. hemiparesis
4. Paralysis on one side of the body	d. aphasia
5. Temporary interruption of the blood flow to part of the brain	e. complete fracture
6. Abnormal movements that are the primary sign of HD	f. pathologic fracture
7. Hip replacement	g. ORIF
8. Pain from an amputation	h. phantom pain
9. Fracture in a diseased bone	i. incomplete fracture
10. Weakness on one side of the body	j. transient ischemic attack
11. Dizziness; spinning sensation	k. vascular
12. Break across the entire cross-section of the bone	l. closed fracture
13. A stroke or brain attack	m. compound fracture
14. Occurs when the skin is intact and not broken	n. THA
15. Occurs when the skin over the fracture is broken	o. hemiplegia
16. Term for an area containing many blood vessels that bleeds readily when a bone is fractured	p. vertigo

Completion

Complete the statements in the spaces provided.

1. Passive range-of-motion exercises _____ and _____.

2. An abnormal shortening and deformity of muscles is called a _____.

3. Moving each toe away from the second toe is called _____.

4. Moving each finger toward the middle finger is called _____.

5. Touching the thumb to the little finger of the same hand is called _____.

6. Rolling the hip in a circular motion toward the midline is called _____.

7. Small fluid-filled sacs found around joints are called _____.

8. Inflammation of a joint is called _____.

9. Any break in the continuity of a bone is a _____.

10. If the broken bone protrudes through the skin, it is called a/an _____ fracture.

11. Traction that uses several weights and lines that are fastened to the outside of the body with a harness-type device is called _____ traction.

12. The pressure of tissue and fluid within the skull is called _____ pressure.

13. Other names for stroke are _____ or cerebrovascular accident.

14. The symptoms of a stroke depend on the area of _____ that becomes ischemic.

15. A stroke on one side of the brain affects function on the _____ side of the body.

16. Post-stroke patients have a high level of _____.

17. Patients with post polio syndrome are very sensitive to _____, particularly in the feet and legs.

18. Patients with post polio syndrome need close _____ after surgery because they commonly experience complications.

19. Amyotrophic lateral sclerosis is a progressive neuromuscular disease that causes muscle weakness and _____.

20. _____ acuity is intact in patients with amyotrophic lateral sclerosis.

21. The most common cause of autonomic dysreflexia is _____.

Short Answer

Briefly answer the following questions.

1. What are three dangers of insufficient exercise?

    a. _____

    b. _____

    c. _____

2. What five special techniques should you use when carrying out ROM exercises?

    a. _____

    b. _____

    c. _____

    d. _____

    e. _____

3. What are five ways to immobilize a fracture?

   a. _____

   b. _____

   c. _____

   d. _____

   e. _____

4. What eight special nursing care procedures must be given to the patient who is in a fresh plaster leg cast?

   a. _____

   b. _____

   c. _____

   d. _____

   e. _____

   f. _____

   g. _____

   h. _____

5. What are four general factors to keep in mind as care is given to the patient who is in traction?

   a. _____

   b. _____

   c. _____

   d. _____

6. Define the following range-of-motion terms.

   a. extension _____

   b. abduction _____

   c. rotation: lateral _____

   d. eversion _____

   e. inversion _____

   f. pronation _____

   g. radial deviation _____

   h. ulnar deviation _____

   i. plantar flexion _____

   j. dorsiflexion _____

7. List two changes that may occur after a cast dries that suggest infection or ulceration under the cast.

   a. _____

   b. _____

8. List six general orders following hip surgery.

a. _____

b. _____

c. _____

d. _____

e. _____

f. _____

9. List four general orders following joint replacement surgery.

a. _____

b. _____

c. _____

d. _____

10. List three benefits of continuous passive motion therapy.

a. _____

b. _____

c. _____

11. List five signs or symptoms of compartment syndrome.

a. _____

b. _____

c. _____

d. _____

e. _____

12. Identify the fractures by writing the proper names in the spaces provided.

a. _____   b. _____

A   B

13. Figures A and B represent two patients who each have a new right hip prosthesis. Identify the incorrect behavior being demonstrated.

a. _____

b. _____

14. List four nursing care measures used in the care of a patient who has had a cerebrovascular accident.

   a. _____

   b. _____

   c. _____

   d. _____

15. List eight signs and symptoms of post polio syndrome.

   a. _____

   b. _____

   c. _____

   d. _____

   e. _____

   f. _____

   g. _____

   h. _____

16. List at least eight conditions that cause autonomic dysreflexia.

a. _____

b. _____

c. _____

d. _____

e. _____

f. _____

g. _____

h. _____

17. List five signs and symptoms of autonomic dysreflexia.

a. _____

b. _____

c. _____

d. _____

e. _____

True/False

Mark the following true or false by circling T or F.

1. T F Patients who are paralyzed are prone to pressure ulcers.

2. T F Parkinson's disease is characterized by muscular rigidity and tremors.

3. T F Tremors of Parkinson's disease become worse when the person is inactive.

4. T F Multiple sclerosis is a progressive disease associated with inadequate levels of neurotransmitters in the cerebellum and brain stem.

5. T F Seizure syndrome is sometimes known as epilepsy.

6. T F Patients with spinal cord injuries need long-term nursing care.

7. T F Meningitis is an inflammation of the inner ear that may result in deafness.

8. T F An aura occurs after a seizure.

9. T F Hemiparesis is paralysis on one side of the body.

10. T F Paraplegia is paralysis below the waist.

Clinical Situations

Briefly describe how a nursing assistant should react to the following situations.

1. The toes of your patient in a leg cast felt cold and looked bluish.

_____

2. Your patient has fibromyalgia. Despite receiving pain medication an hour ago, she is crying and says she has severe pain.

_____

_____

3. You find Mr. Lossero, an 82-year-old confused patient, on the floor. His right leg is shortened and externally rotated.

_____

_____

_____

4. Mrs. Huynh has a short leg cast, which is dry. She has an order to take a shower.

_____

_____

5. Your patient has a fractured tibia and fractured radius. Both extremities are casted in plaster casts. You enter the room and the patient tells you the pain in her tibia is agonizing—even worse than it was when she fell and broke it.

_____

_____

_____

6. Your patient complained of discomfort during range-of-motion exercises.

_____

_____

_____

7. The patient has had a lower leg amputated below the knee. You must position the extremity.

_____

_____

_____

8. You notice a change in the level of consciousness of your patient who has a head injury.

_____

_____

_____

9. Your patient in the private room has post polio syndrome. The bed is on the opposite wall of the room from her bed at home. She is having trouble getting into and out of bed.

_____

_____

_____

10. Mr. Herrera, an ALS patient, had difficulty swallowing his regular diet when you fed him. He kept coughing and choking.

_____

_____

_____

RELATING TO THE NURSING PROCESS

Write the step of the nursing process that is related to the nursing assistant action.

Nursing Assistant Action	Nursing Process Step
1. The nursing assistant handles the wet cast with open palms.	_____
2. The nursing assistant supports above and below the joint being exercised.	_____
3. The nursing assistant stops carrying out range of motion and reports to the nurse when the patient complains of pain.	_____
4. The nursing assistant carries out each ROM exercise five times.	_____
5. The nursing assistant reports the patient's feelings of numbness in the toes of the newly casted leg.	_____
6. The nursing assistant helps support the patient in a spica cast while another assistant changes the linen.	_____
7. The nursing assistant is very careful not to disturb the weights while caring for the patient using skeletal traction.	_____
8. The nursing assistant asks the nursing supervisor to review the traction lines on the skeletal traction before she begins to give care.	_____
9. The nursing assistant notes uncontrolled body movements in the patient who has a head injury and calls this to the nurse's attention.	_____
10. The nursing assistant helps the nurse turn and position the patient who has had a stroke.	_____
11. The nursing assistant finds a patient who is convulsing. She calls for help but does not leave the patient alone.	_____
12. The nursing assistant pays particular attention when the patient with Parkinson's disease ambulates, knowing that he is more apt to fall.	_____

Caring for Patients with Disorders of the Sensory Organs

OBJECTIVES

After completing this unit, you will be able to:

- Spell and define terms.
- Identify aging changes of the sensory organs.
- Describe common disorders of the sensory organs.
- Describe nursing assistant actions and observations related to the care of patients with disorders of the sensory organs.
- Explain the proper care, handling, and insertion of a hearing aid.
- Demonstrate Procedures 92 and 93 (set out in this unit in the textbook).

UNIT SUMMARY

The human body is controlled by the nervous system. The sensory organs are part of the nervous system, and provide sensations related to seeing, hearing, touching, tasting, and smelling.

The sensory organs need very little stimulation before the person notices sensations. This remarkable system acts by sending messages to and from the brain in response to signals transmitted to the body from the environment. The nervous system controls sensation by noticing a stimulation, sending a message to the brain for interpretation of the message, then sending a message through the nerves back to the body describing how to respond to the message. This process occurs very rapidly—usually in a split second. A disorder of the sensory system can affect many other body systems.

Nursing assistants use their sensory organs when making observations, identifying problems, and noting changes in condition.

- Like other systems, the sensory system changes with age. As a person ages, normal body changes increase the reaction time. The result is that more sensory input is needed before the person becomes aware of incoming sensations. Some aging changes can be corrected, but the improvement may not seem as good as the senses the person remembers from his or her younger years.

- The eyes provide information to the brain for interpretation and action. The eye changes shape slightly to meet various visual needs.

- The ears affect hearing and balance.

- The senses of smell and taste are closely related. These sensations affect safety and food enjoyment.

- About 20 different types of touch nerve endings send messages to the brain. The most sensitive areas of the body are the hands, lips, face, neck, tongue, fingertips, and feet. The least sensitive part of the body is the middle of the back. Humans have more pain receptors than any other type. Pain serves as a warning that something is wrong.

NURSING ASSISTANT ALERT

Action	Benefit
Be consistent in care and use established routines.	Requires fewer stressful adjustments for the patient.
Use your sensations to identify changes (improvements or deterioration) in patients' conditions.	Ensures quality care because changes are identified and acted upon in a timely manner.
Report and document observations and care accurately.	Ensures timely response and nursing intervention. Provides a database for correct nursing evaluations and interventions.
Follow care plan instructions for management of prostheses and sensory aids.	Provides adaptive devices and/or appliances to help compensate for sensory organ dysfunction.

ACTIVITIES

Vocabulary Exercise

Complete the crossword puzzle by using the definitions provided.

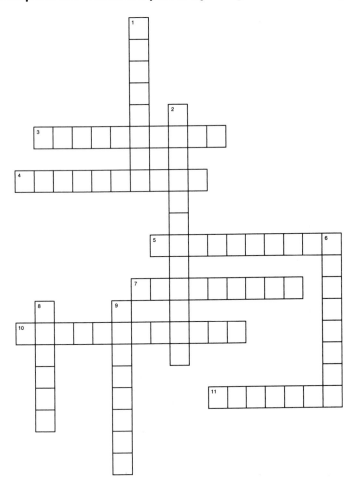

Across

3 A person with a vision or hearing _____ may need a corrective device, such as glasses or a hearing aid, to compensate for reduced sensory function.

4 Warm or cool _____ are used as a treatment for dry, itchy eyes.

5 An _____ eye is used for cosmetic purposes when a person's eye has been removed.

7 Clouding of the lens of the eyes

10 A progressive form of deafness of unknown cause

11 A system of raised dots that are read by using the sense of touch

Down

1 _____ disease results from fluid buildup in the inner ear, and can affect both hearing and balance.

2 Macular _____ is a breakdown of the retina that occurs over a long period of time.

6 Sign _____ is one method of communicating with patients who are deaf.

8 _____ media is an infection of the middle ear.

9 Increased pressure in the eye

Completion

Complete the following statements in the spaces provided.

1. _____ are the leading cause of vision loss in older adults.

2. The person with _____ experiences decreased vision and gradual loss of peripheral vision.

3. The incidence of macular degeneration increases with _____.

4. An eye _____ is usually inserted after surgical removal of an eye.

5. Following cataract surgery, the patient should avoid _____.

6. Following cataract surgery, it is especially important to report _____ or _____ in the operative eye.

7. If it is to remain out of the socket, store an artificial eye in a marked cup in _____ or _____.

8. When inserting an artificial eye, position the notched edge of the eye _____.

9. Otitis media is an infection of the _____ and may result in _____ of the ossicles, leading to deafness.

10. It is important not to let a hearing aid get _____.

11. In a patient with glaucoma, the pressure is _____ within the eye.

12. _____ protects the inner ears.

13. Shave the patient who uses a hearing aid with an electric razor _____ inserting the hearing aid.

14. Most tastes originate with _____.

15. Of the five senses, the sense of _____ is the weakest.

16. Each fingertip contains approximately _____ touch receptors.

17. In addition to providing information that something is wrong, the pain receptors also provide important information related to _____ and _____.

18. _____ is a disorder of the inner ear that can affect hearing and balance, and cause dizziness, vertigo, tinnitus, vomiting, and the sensation of fullness in the ear.

19. Store a hearing aid at _____ when it is not being worn.

20. The minimum amount of stimulation required for a person to notice a sensation is the _____.

Short Answer

Briefly answer the following questions.

1. List six aging changes to the eyes.

   a. _____

   b. _____

   c. _____

   d. _____

   e. _____

   f. _____

2. List four aging changes to the ears.

a. _____

b. _____

c. _____

d. _____

3. In addition to routine postoperative care and vital sign monitoring, list five nursing assistant measures to take in the care of patients with cataract surgery.

a. _____

b. _____

c. _____

d. _____

e. _____

4. List five nursing assistant measures to take in the care of patients with glaucoma.

a. _____

b. _____

c. _____

d. _____

e. _____

True/False

Mark the following true or false by circling T or F.

1.   T   F   Dehydration may be a problem if the area between the patient's gums and cheeks is dry, even if the patient is a mouth breather.

2.   T   F   Taste buds decrease in number as part of normal aging.

3.   T   F   Nearsightedness occurs when the eye is too short.

4.   T   F   The shape of the ear may change, so a hearing aid may have to be refitted.

5.   T   F   Remove ear wax regularly with cotton swabs.

6.   T   F   Some medical problems cause a decreased sense of smell and loss of awareness of unpleasant odors.

7.   T   F   Saliva production increases with age.

8.   T   F   Cataract surgery is an outpatient procedure.

9.   T   F   Women blink about twice as much as men.

10. T   F   Patients who are legally blind have no vision.

11. T   F   A hearing aid is a relatively inexpensive device.

12. T   F   Fluid and pus form within the outer ear canal when a patient has otitis media.

RELATING TO THE NURSING PROCESS

Write the step of the nursing process that is related to the nursing assistant action.

Nursing Assistant Action   **Nursing Process Step**

1. The nursing assistant informs the nurse that Mr. Lockhart's eyes are red and flaky in appearance, and he is rubbing them frequently.   _____

2. After giving three days of warm compress treatments, the nursing assistant informs the nurse that Mr. Lockhart's eyes are less red and he has stopped rubbing them.   _____

3. The nursing assistant monitors Mr. Hoyer's postoperative vital signs and clips the call light to the sheet next to his hand after cataract surgery.   _____

4. The nursing assistant arranges her assignment so she has extra time to spend with Joseph Mahoney, a patient who is completely deaf and blind.   _____

5. The nursing assistant reminds Mr. Hoyer not to rub his eyes postoperatively.   _____

6. The nursing assistant removes Mrs. Nuñez's artificial eye and soaks it in the solution listed on the care plan.   _____

7. The nursing assistant notifies the nurse that Mrs. Nuñez has yellow drainage in the socket behind her artificial eye.   _____

8. The nursing assistant asks the nurse for instructions on removing ear wax and cleaning Mr. Heaney's hearing aid.   _____

DEVELOPING GREATER INSIGHT

Complete the following statements to show your understanding of communication with patients who have sensory impairments.

1. When communicating with a patient who is hard of hearing:

   Make sure the patient can _____ you.

   Stand on the patient's _____ side.

   Do not _____ your mouth when speaking.

   Speak _____, distinctly, and naturally.

   Use _____ gestures and body language to help express your meaning.

2. When communicating with a patient who is visually impaired:

   Describe the environment and _____ around the patient to establish a frame of reference.

   Touch the patient _____ on the hand to avoid startling him or her.

   Be _____ when giving directions.

   When entering a room, _____ yourself and state your purpose.

   Assist the patient to use _____ books, if desired.

Caring for Patients with Disorders of the Endocrine and Reproductive Systems

After completing this unit, you will be able to:

- Spell and define terms.

- Identify aging changes of the endocrine and reproductive systems.

- Recognize the signs and symptoms of hypoglycemia and hyperglycemia.

- Describe nursing assistant actions and observations related to the care of patients with disorders of the endocrine and reproductive systems.

- Perform Procedures 94 and 95 (set out in this unit in the textbook).

UNIT SUMMARY

- The endocrine system coordinates, regulates, and controls body functions through the use of chemical messengers called *hormones*. Hormones travel about in the body through the bloodstream.

- Common conditions of the endocrine system are those involving the thyroid gland, reproductive organs, adrenal glands, and reproductive organs. Fluid balance in the body is also partially regulated by the endocrine system.

- Diabetes mellitus is a chronic disease that results from a deficiency of insulin or a resistance to the effects of insulin. In this condition, the body cannot properly process food into energy. This endocrine system disorder requires close monitoring and care. In the United States, 20.8 million

people (7% of the population) had diabetes by 2005. Diabetes occurs in people of all ages and races, and the incidence increases with age.

- The functions of the reproductive system are gender-specific. This system works closely with the endocrine system, through use of hormones, to control body function and secondary sex characteristics.

- Practicing proper infection control is essential when caring for patients who have disorders of the endocrine and reproductive systems, as bloodborne pathogens and sexually transmitted diseases can be readily transmitted through blood, body fluids, mucous membranes, and body secretions.

NURSING ASSISTANT ALERT

Action	Benefit
Follow orders and report the patient's response.	Helps those who are hormonally imbalanced to become stabilized.
Pay close attention to the diabetic's feet and dietary intake.	Contributes to foot health and proper blood sugar levels.
Perform various diabetes testing procedures; recognize and report abnormal values.	Ensures tight blood sugar control and reduces the risk of complications.
Know the signs and symptoms of diabetic coma and insulin shock and report them promptly.	Early intervention can prevent development of serious complications.
Be alert to and report indications of infections or abnormalities of the reproductive tract.	Starting therapy early can avert more extensive body damage.
Recognize that any threat to the reproductive organs has a strong psychological impact on an individual.	Provides strong patient support.

ACTIVITIES

Vocabulary Exercise

Find the following words in the puzzle. *Words in parentheses are not in the puzzle.* In the space provided, write a definition of each word.

h	z	C	e	n	o	t	e	c	a	F	h
w	y	O	s	e	p	r	e	H	S	y	p
b	f	p	v	Y	t	T	p	B	p	S	r
s	n	t	e	J	d	o	S	o	p	v	o
e	i	e	u	r	X	m	g	j	V	e	l
t	l	t	t	P	t	l	m	k	w	h	a
e	u	a	t	t	y	r	O	t	C	c	p
b	s	n	T	c	l	m	o	e	r	u	s
a	n	y	e	g	t	D	l	p	D	o	s
i	i	m	l	a	n	c	e	t	h	d	Z
d	i	a	e	r	c	n	a	h	c	y	E
a	z	H	a	e	h	r	r	o	n	o	g

1. acetone

_____

2. chancre

_____

3. diabetes (mellitus)

_____

4. douche

_____

5. FSBS

_____

6. gonorrhea

_____

7. herpes (simplex II)

_____

8. hypertrophy

_____

9. hypoglycemia

_____

10. insulin

_____

11. lancet

_____

12. (uterine) prolapse

_____

13. tetany

_____

Short Answer

Define the following terms or abbreviations in the spaces provided.

1. Addison's disease

_____

2. brachytherapy

_____

3. Cushing's syndrome

_____

4. glucose

_____

5. hyperglycemia

_____

6. hypersecretion

_____

7. hyperthyroidism

_____

8. hyposecretion

_____

9. hypothyroidism

_____

10. insulin-dependent diabetes mellitus (IDDM)

_____

11. metabolism rate

_____

12. non–insulin-dependent diabetes mellitus (NIDDM)

_____

13. prostatectomy

_____

14. sexually transmitted disease (STD)

_____

15. simple goiter

_____

16. syphilis

_____

Completion

Complete the following statements in the spaces provided.

1. The role of glands in the body is to secrete _____.

2. The chemicals secreted by glands _____ body activities and growth.

3. A major contribution the nursing assistant can make to the care of a patient with hyperthyroidism is to keep the room _____ and be patient and calm.

4. The person with hyperthyroidism is at high risk for _____ due to rapid metabolism.

5. The patient who has had a thyroidectomy should be monitored for a severe, acute muscle spasm called _____.

6. Hypersecretion of adrenal cortical hormones causes a disease syndrome called _____.

7. The patient with Addison's disease may become dehydrated and has a low tolerance to _____.

8. The normal fasting blood glucose range is between _____ and _____.

9. Two medications given for diabetes mellitus are insulin and _____ drugs.

10. A patient with diabetes has a sweet, fruity odor to his breath, so you might suspect _____.

11. A patient with diabetes is feeling excited, nervous, and hungry, so you might suspect _____.

12. Take special care of the _____ of the patient who has diabetes.

13. Daily foot care for the diabetic includes carefully _____ and _____ the feet.

14. Do not allow _____ to collect between the toes of a person who has diabetes.

15. Diabetic patients should never be permitted to go _____.

16. A common enlargement of the prostate gland is called benign _____.

17. The tube-like organ passing through the center of the prostate gland is the _____.

18. A major problem for men suffering from the condition named in question 16 is urinary
_____.

19. A patient with a nursing diagnosis of *Disturbed Body Image* will probably need a great deal of
_____.

20. If untreated, syphilis passes through _____ stages.

21. An outbreak of herpes may be preceded by _____, _____,
and _____.

22. Hypoglycemia related to diabetes may also be called _____ or _____.

23. The fluid inside the blisters associated with genital herpes is _____.

24. The blisters associated with genital herpes will heal in about _____.

25. A person with genital herpes may _____ even when an outbreak is not present.

26. Herpes is caused by a _____.

27. Herpes simplex II is transmitted primarily through _____.

28. Tertiary syphilis is not _____.

Short Answer

Briefly answer the following questions.

1. List four factors that can contribute to a hypoglycemic state.

   a. _____

   b. _____

   c. _____

   d. _____

2. List four signs and symptoms of a hypoglycemic state.

   a. _____

   b. _____

   c. _____

   d. _____

3. List five nursing assistant responsibilities in caring for a patient who has diabetes mellitus.

a. _____

b. _____

c. _____

d. _____

4. List 10 signs and symptoms of sexually transmitted disease.

a. _____

b. _____

c. _____

d. _____

e. _____

f. _____

g. _____

h. _____

i. _____

j. _____

5. Compare the signs and symptoms of diabetic coma and insulin shock.

	Diabetic Coma	Insulin Shock
Respirations		
Pulse		
Skin		

RELATING TO THE NURSING PROCESS

Write the step of the nursing process that is related to the nursing assistant action.

Nursing Assistant Action   **Nursing Process Step**

1. The nursing assistant reports that her patient, a diabetic, has diarrhea.   _____

2. The nursing assistant makes sure the room of the patient with hyperthyroidism is kept cool and quiet.   _____

3. The nursing assistant documents the amount of fluid the patient with diabetes is consuming.   _____

4. The nursing assistant reports that the patient with diabetes has pale, moist skin and seems nervous.   _____

5. The nursing assistant tests the patient's urine for acetone using the Ketostix strip test.   _____

6. The nursing assistant carefully washes and inspects the feet of the patient with diabetes daily.   _____

7. The nursing assistant reports to the nurse that the patient is complaining of itching and has a watery vaginal discharge.   _____

8. The nursing assistant checks for bleeding after the patient has had a mastectomy.   _____

9. The nursing assistant informs the nurse of the grief and frustrations the postoperative mastectomy patient is expressing.   _____

10. The nursing assistant inserts the douche nozzle slowly, while the fluid is flowing, in an upward and backward motion.   _____

11. The nursing assistant carefully notes and reports color and amount of drainage from all areas for the patient who has had a prostatectomy.   _____

12. The nursing assistant reports that the patient's postoperative mastectomy dressing is saturated with blood, and the nurse changes it. The nursing assistant rechecks the dressing and notes that it has only a tiny spot on it. He informs the nurse that the patient is having less drainage than previously.   _____

DEVELOPING GREATER INSIGHT

Circle the correct alternative in the following statements.

Situation for questions 1 through 6: The CDC have documented the transmission of hepatitis B infection through the use of community (shared) glucose meters. In addition to hepatitis B, sharing of meters holds the potential for transmitting other types of infections.

1. Hepatitis B and other bloodborne pathogens (are stable and can survive) (are unstable and will die quickly) on environmental surfaces and equipment at room temperature.

2. Bloodborne pathogens (can) (cannot) be transmitted on contaminated environmental surfaces and equipment.

3. To reduce the risk of infection, (wipe the blood glucose meter with disinfectant) (wash the blood glucose meter well in hot, soapy water).

4. Clean the blood glucose meter (after each use) (at the end of the shift).

5. Disinfect the spring-loaded lancet holder (after each use) (at the end of the shift).

6. Discard used lancets in the (sharps container) (trash can).

7. Oral herpes and genital herpes are caused by (different pathogens) (the same organism).

8. Touching a cold sore on the mouth, then touching the genital area (will) (will not) transmit the herpes to the genitalia, and vice versa.

9. The causative agent for herpes (leaves the body) (becomes dormant) when signs and symptoms of infection subside.

10. Herpes (can) (cannot) be passed to another person when no lesions are present.

11. An active herpes lesion (is) (is not) painful.

12. People with the herpes infection generally have (one episode) (repeated episodes).

13. One in (five) (fifty) American adults has genital herpes.

14. A person with genital herpes (will know of the infection) (may not know of the infection).

15. Medication for herpes (eliminates the infection) (relieves the symptoms).

Expanded Role of the Nursing Assistant

U N I T **40**

Caring for Obstetrical Patients and Neonates

OBJECTIVES

After completing this unit, you will be able to:

- Spell and define terms.
- Define *doula* and identify the role and responsibilities of the doula as a member of the childbirth team.
- Assist in care of the normal postpartum patient.
- Properly change a perineal pad.
- Recognize reportable observations of patients in the postpartum period.
- Assist in care of the normal newborn.
- Demonstrate three methods of safely holding a baby.
- Describe nursing assistant actions and observations related to the care of the newborn infant.
- List measures to prevent inadvertent switching, misidentification, and abduction of infants.
- Assist in carrying out the discharge procedures for mother and infant.
- Demonstrate Procedures 96–106 (set out in this unit in the textbook).

UNIT SUMMARY

The care of the obstetrical patient is a very specialized area of medicine. It includes:

- Supervision of the mother during the labor and delivery and postpartum periods to discharge.

- Care of the neonate.

The nursing assistant may participate in this care under the close direction of the professional staff. A thorough understanding of your responsibilities and close attention to the details of care help ensure a successful and safe hospital stay.

You must get advanced training and supervision before you attempt to perform the procedures presented in this unit. In addition, you may perform them only with proper authorization and under proper supervision.

NURSING ASSISTANT ALERT

Action	Benefit
Follow orders carefully during the delivery and postpartum periods.	Helps ensure a successful and safe pregnancy and delivery.
Handle and carry babies securely in an approved manner.	Protects the baby from injury.
Be open with and supportive of parents.	Provides essential emotional support when parents need it the most.
Practice and teach safety and infection control.	Helps ensure positive outcomes and prevents injuries and infections.

ACTIVITIES

Vocabulary Exercise

Each line has four different spellings of a word. Circle the correctly spelled word.

1. lokia	lochia	logia	lochea
2. neonat	nionat	nionate	neonate
3. fetal	fetle	fietal	fetyl
4. epescotomy	episiotomy	epysiotomy	episiotomie
5. umbalical	umbilicle	umbilical	umbelical
6. placenta	placentar	placenter	plecentar
7. sircumsition	circumsishun	searcumcision	circumcision
8. amneotac	amniotic	ammneotic	amneottec
9. postpartim	postpartem	postpartum	postpartam
10. stattis	stattes	statas	status
11. doola	doula	dulla	dooluh
12. foarskin	foursken	foreskin	fourschin

ACTIVITIES

Vocabulary Exercise

In the figure, put a circle around the word defined.

a	p	e	t	t	e	l	o	s	i	n
u	l	o	l	o	c	h	i	a	o	a
n	e	u	s	h	m	w	g	i	e	t
o	t	c	o	t	s	o	t	b	p	n
i	a	b	g	d	p	u	f	a	l	e
t	n	u	l	r	l	a	h	b	o	c
c	o	x	u	o	a	i	r	d	c	a
u	e	h	v	r	u	c	g	t	c	l
d	n	n	b	s	a	l	t	c	u	p
b	i	u	g	n	i	p	r	u	b	m
a	r	d	e	l	i	v	e	r	y	j

1. The process in which the uterus returns to its normal size

2. The care of the mother after delivery

3. Removing an infant from the unit or facility without permission

4. The _____ room is the area where infants are born.

5. A closed crib used to keep the infant warm

6. The tissue attached to the mother's uterine wall, to which the umbilical cord is attached

7. Method of assisting an infant to expel air swallowed during feeding

8. Name for the postdelivery vaginal discharge

9. Mother's helper

10. Term to describe red color of vaginal discharge

11. Term for the newly born infant

Completion

Complete the following statements in the spaces provided.

1. The fetus in the uterus receives nourishment through the _____.

2. The afterbirth is called the _____.

3. While weighing a baby, keep one _____ over the baby at all times.

4. If it is necessary to carry an infant in your arms, always _____ through a doorway.

5. Never turn your _____ when the infant is on an unprotected surface.

6. Be sure to wash hands _____ and _____ handling each child and after each _____ change.

7. A circumcision should be checked _____.

8. The baby is dressed in _____ clothes for discharge.

9. The "cramping" mothers feel postpartum is due to the uterus _____.

10. When removing a soiled perineal pad, always wear _____ and fold the soiled side of the pad _____.

11. Teach the mother to handle the pad _____.

12. Teach the mother to cleanse the perineum from _____ to _____.

13. Mothers who are breast-feeding should be instructed to wash their breasts using a _____ motion from _____ outward.

14. The baby must be kept warm until his _____ stabilizes.

15. In the nursery, the _____, weight, and vital signs are measured.

16. The _____ is a member of the childbirth team who is responsible for supporting and comforting the mother, and for facilitating and enhancing communication between the mother and medical professionals.

17. Gently stroke the infant's _____ to get the baby to open the mouth and turn toward the breast.

18. Upon admission to the nursery, the infant's _____ temperature is monitored and recorded every _____ to _____ minutes until stable.

19. When lifting an infant, always support the _____.

20. Cover the infant's head with a _____ to prevent loss of _____.

21. Advise the mother to press and hold the breast back, if necessary, so it _____.

22. A normal newborn will urinate _____ to _____ times a day.

23. The infant's first stools are _____ in color. Over the next few days, the color changes to _____, then to _____.

24. The infant's length is measured with the infant in the _____ position.

25. The infant's admission bath is given after _____.

26. Elimination is _____ and the _____ of stool documented.

Short Answer

Briefly answer the following questions.

1. What is meant when we say that the length of pregnancy is divided into three trimesters?

_____

_____

_____

2. List two responsibilities of the doula.

   a. _____

   b. _____

3. What three techniques might be ordered to relieve the perineal discomfort of an episiotomy?

   a. _____

   b. _____

   c. _____

4. List two methods of measuring an infant.

   a. _____

   b. _____

5. How should the baby be lifted from the crib?

   a. _____

   b. _____

Clinical Situations

Briefly explain how the nursing assistant should react to the following situations.

1. The mother of an infant tells you she feels offended when you wear gloves when assisting with breast-feeding and changing the infant after eating. How can you tactfully tell her why gloves are necessary?

_____

_____

2. Your facility policy states that the length of an infant must be measured twice. The measurements must be within 1/8 inch of each other. Why is this done?

_____

_____

RELATING TO THE NURSING PROCESS

Write the step of the nursing process that is related to the nursing assistant action.

Nursing Assistant Action   **Nursing Process Step**

1. The nursing assistant weighs patients and measures vital signs.   _____

2. The nursing assistant helps other staff members transfer the newly delivered mother from stretcher to bed.   _____

3. The nursing assistant checks the mother's vital signs as ordered following a cesarean section.   _____

4. The nursing assistant measures and records the first postpartum voiding.   _____

5. The nursing assistant instructs the mother to stand up before flushing the toilet.   _____

6. The nursing assistant immediately reports to the nurse when she finds the uterus of the new postpartum patient becoming soft and enlarged.   _____

7. Mrs. Ehlers has been having very heavy vaginal drainage. The nursing assistant helps the patient to change a saturated peri pad at 2:00 PM. She returns to the room at 2:30 PM to see if the patient's vaginal flow has subsided.   _____

8. The nursing assistant reorganizes her priorities so she can spend time with a patient who has been crying.   _____

Rehabilitation and Restorative Services

OBJECTIVES

After completing this unit, you will be able to:

- Spell and define terms.
- Compare and contrast rehabilitation and restorative nursing care.
- Describe the role of the nursing assistant in rehabilitation and restorative care.
- Describe the principles of rehabilitation.
- List the elements of successful rehabilitation/restorative care.
- List six complications resulting from inactivity.
- Describe four approaches used for restorative programs.
- List guidelines for providing restorative care.
- Describe monitoring of the patient's response to care.

UNIT SUMMARY

Rehabilitation and restorative care are designed to help patients reach an optimal level of personal ability. The most successful programs:

- Begin as soon as possible
- Stress abilities
- Treat the whole patient

Rehabilitation and restorative care provide patients with life skills that they will use regularly. They do not include "busy work," or provide skills the patient is not likely to need or use.

Care is planned by an interdisciplinary health care team, of which the nursing assistant is an important member. Nursing assistants participate in the restorative program by:

- Knowing and following the stated nursing health care plan
- Supporting the patient's efforts toward independence
- Assisting the nurses with procedures designed to meet specific patient needs and goals
- Maintaining the patient's nutrition

Nursing assistants can make a valuable contribution to the success of the patient's program by demonstrating a consistent, positive, and patient attitude.

NURSING ASSISTANT ALERT

Action	Benefit
Give patient opportunities to make decisions whenever possible.	Adds to patient's sense of control.
Treat patient with dignity at all times.	Encourages patient's self-esteem and fosters attitude of cooperation.
Be encouraging and give praise.	Promotes positive attitude in patient and inspires patient to keep trying.
Know the care plan and follow it.	Assures that restorative/rehabilitation program will be focused and consistent.

ACTIVITIES

Vocabulary Exercise

Using the definitions, write the proper words in the spaces provided.

1. A disability that prevents a person from fulfilling a role that is normal for that person
   _____

2. Physician who specializes in rehabilitation _____

3. Ordinary items that are modified for a specific patient _____

4. Process that assists the patient to reach an optimal level of ability _____

5. Impairment that affects the person's ability to perform an activity that a person of that age would usually be able to do _____

Completion

Complete the following statements in the spaces provided. Select the proper terms from the list provided.

care	disability	disease or injury	handicap
influence	optimum level of performance	problems	rehabilitation
retraining	same approach	self-care deficit	strength

1. Rehabilitation refers to a process in which the patient strives for the _____.

2. A person with paralysis suffers from a _____.

3. A person who has been in bed for a long time because of heart disease may require _____.

4. All the different disciplines that are involved in rehabilitation work together to resolve _____ and plan _____.

5. Any activity a patient is capable of doing is considered a _____.

6. Patients and family _____ the emotional and mental health of patients who are being rehabilitated.

7. A patient who cannot complete any or all of the ADLs independently is said to have a _____.

8. Damage to the brain usually occurs because of _____.

9. Restorative programs are sometimes referred to as _____ programs.

10. It is important that everyone working with a patient in restorative care use the _____.

Short Answer

Briefly answer the following questions.

1. List five common goals of rehabilitation and restorative nursing.

   a. _____

   b. _____

   c. _____

   d. _____

   e. _____

2. State seven activities that are included in the tasks of daily living (ADLs).

   a. _____

   b. _____

   c. _____

   d. _____

   e. _____

   f. _____

   g. _____

3. List three interdisciplinary rehabilitation goals for a patient with a disability.

   a. _____

   b. _____

   c. _____

4. Name five professionals, other than nurses and physicians, who are involved in the rehabilitative process.

   a. _____

   b. _____

   c. _____

   d. _____

   e. _____

5. Write the four principles that form the foundation for successful rehabilitation or restorative care.

   a. _____

   b. _____

   c. _____

   d. _____

6. Name four approaches used in restorative programs.

   a. _____

   b. _____

   c. _____

   d. _____

7. Describe the type of environment that benefits patients and promotes success in a restorative program.

   _____

   _____

Clinical Situations

Briefly describe how a nursing assistant should react to the following situations.

1. Mr. Fronzoni is very frustrated as the nursing assistant explains how to put his socks on before the shoes.
   _____
   _____

2. Mr. Tracy has a roommate who repeatedly interrupts as the nursing assistant tries to help Mr. Tracy hold his glass. _____
   _____

3. Mrs. Davis is frustrated this morning and says that her progress is "just too slow."
   _____
   _____

4. The nursing assistant is assigned for the first time this morning to care for Mrs. Washington, who needs help with her self-feeding program. _____
   _____
   _____

5. Mr. Smythe is left-handed and has an adaptive device for his left hand. The device is on his bedside table as he attempts to brush his teeth. _____
   _____

6. Mrs. Missel is unable to gather the necessary equipment to give herself a bath and then carry out the procedure.
   _____
   _____

7. Ms. Wexford has difficulty manipulating her clothing when she uses the toilet. She is able to stand and sit independently. _____
   _____

8. Mr. Surgeant can hold his toothbrush and put it in his mouth, but then just holds it there.
   _____
   _____

9. Mrs. Malone is in a restorative program in the skilled care facility, but seems bored and restless between activity sessions. _____
   _____

10. Complete the chart by placing an *X* in the appropriate column.

> Mr. Cochran is admitted for rehabilitation. Mr. Ward is admitted to the same skilled care facility, but his goal is restoration. How does rehabilitation differ from restoration?

Activity	Rehabilitation	Restoration
a. OBRA rules require all skilled care facilities to provide this service.	_____	_____
b. Goal is to increase the patient's quality of life.	_____	_____
c. May be provided in a general acute care hospital.	_____	_____
d. Usually more aggressive and intense.	_____	_____
e. Slower therapies over weeks, months, or indefinitely.	_____	_____
f. Requires the skills of many different therapists.	_____	_____
g. Primarily a nursing responsibility, with consultation.	_____	_____

RELATING TO THE NURSING PROCESS

Write the step of the nursing process that is related to the nursing assistant action.

Nursing Assistant Action	Nursing Process Step
1. The nursing assistant begins passive exercises and positioning for Mrs. Burton, who is stable after a right-sided stroke.	_____
2. The nursing assistant encourages Mr. Jackson, who has poor strength in his dominant right hand, as he tries to feed himself with his left hand.	_____
3. The nursing assistant participates in team care conferences.	_____
4. The nursing assistant reports that Mrs. Parson is able to move her hands but is unable to select and hold items.	_____

Response to Basic Emergencies

Response to Basic Emergencies

OBJECTIVES

After completing this unit, you will be able to:

- Spell and define terms.
- Recognize emergency situations that require urgent care.
- Evaluate situations and determine the actions to be taken.
- List and describe the 11 standardized codes.
- Describe how to maintain the patient's airway and breathing.
- Recognize the need for CPR.
- List the benefits of early defibrillation.
- Identify the signs, symptoms, and treatment of common emergency situations.
- Demonstrate Procedures 107–114 (set out in this unit in the textbook).

UNIT SUMMARY

Emergency situations can occur without warning at any time. A person who has been specially trained in the techniques of first aid can be of great service.

- Remain calm.
- Know the correct standardized code words to use to get the correct type of response.

- Remain with the patient (unless otherwise instructed) until further help arrives, and perform any emergency procedures that you are qualified and permitted to do.

- Never overestimate your abilities.

- Use the special skills you have been taught wisely.

Special training will enable you to assess injuries and know the proper steps to follow in:

- Calling for help

- Carrying out lifesaving skills such as CPR

- Controlling bleeding

- Helping victims of disease and trauma

NURSING ASSISTANT ALERT

Action	Benefit
Never overestimate your abilities.	Prevents injuries due to improper actions.
Perform only approved actions.	Can be lifesaving. Avoids legal liability.

ACTIVITIES

Vocabulary Exercise

Complete the puzzle by filling in the missing letters of words found in this unit. Use the definitions to help you discover these words.

1. _ _ _ U _ _   1. Injury

2. _ _ R _ _ _ _   2. Stoppage of heartbeat

3. _ _ _ _ _ _ _ G   3. Sudden loss of consciousness

4. _ _ _ _ _ E _ _   4. An unintended occurrence

5. _ _ _ _ _ _ N _ _   5. A situation that develops rapidly and unexpectedly

6. _ _ _ _ T _ _ _ _ _   6. Emergency cardiac condition

7. _ _ _ _ C _   7. Disturbance of oxygen supply to the tissues and return of blood to the heart

8. _ _ _ _ A _ _   8. To raise

9. _ _ R   9. Cardiopulmonary resuscitation

10. _ E _ _ _ _ _ _ _ _   10. Loss of blood

Completion

Complete the statements in the spaces provided.

1. Your actions should never place the victim in additional _____.

2. First aid techniques are taught as a specific course by the _____.

3. Certification in CPR is provided in courses by the _____ and the American Red Cross.

4. In an emergency situation, always defer to someone who has greater _____ or _____.

5. When you provide first aid, you must deal with the victim's _____ as well as the victim's physical injuries.

6. The first step when arriving at the scene of an accident is to _____ the situation.

7. If you are in a medical facility when an accident occurs, you should _____ for help and keep the patient _____.

8. The national number for emergency help is _____.

9. The most common cause of airway obstruction is _____, so pulling the _____ forward often opens the airway.

10. If oxygen is denied to the body, the most sensitive organ, the _____, may suffer permanent damage.

11. The compression-to-ventilation ratio for CPR is _____ compressions to _____ ventilations.

12. Care that must be given immediately to prevent loss of life is called _____.

13. When moving a victim, always move him as a single _____.

14. The Heimlich maneuver refers to the technique of performing _____ thrusts.

15. Finger sweeps should only be used if you can _____ a foreign body in the victim's throat or mouth.

16. A disturbance of the oxygen supply to the tissues and return of blood to the heart is called _____.

17. The victim who is in shock should be kept _____ down.

18. The loss of heart function is called _____.

19. Seizures do not always follow the same _____.

20. In a generalized tonic-clonic (grand mal) seizure, the patient must be protected against _____ himself.

21. Following a generalized tonic-clonic (grand mal) seizure, the patient may be _____ and _____ for a time and feel very tired.

22. A good way to move a victim of electric shock away from the source of electricity is to use something made of _____.

Short Answer

Briefly answer the following questions.

1. What four basic actions should be taken in all emergency situations?

    a. _____

    b. _____

    c. _____

    d. _____

2. What two types of care are included in first aid?

    a. _____

    b. _____

3. What is the purpose of having standardized code words?

    a. _____

    b. _____

    c. _____

    d. _____

4. What are four ways to summon help for an accident victim in a health facility?

    a. _____

    b. _____

    c. _____

    d. _____

5. How should you check for breathing activity?

    a. _____

    b. _____

6. What order of victim's responses should be checked when providing urgent care?

    a. _____

    b. _____

    c. _____

    d. _____

    e. _____

7. How would you describe the distress signals of choking?

_____

8. What steps should you follow to prevent additional blood loss in a bleeding victim?

    a. _____

    b. _____

    c. _____

    d. _____

    e. _____

    f. _____

9. What are the early signs of shock?

    a. _____

    b. _____

    c. _____

    d. _____

    e. _____

10. What signs and symptoms might indicate that the victim is having a heart attack?

    a. _____

    b. _____

    c. _____

    d. _____

    e. _____

Clinical Situations

Briefly describe how a nursing assistant should react to the following situations.

1. You are the first person on the scene of an auto accident. One person has been thrown out of the car and is lying beside the car, which is on fire. Describe your first action.

_____

_____

2. You discover the husband of your home client on the floor of the basement near a frayed electrical wire. What is your first action?

_____

_____

3. You are in a dining area when an ambulatory patient grasps his throat and is unable to speak.

_____

_____

RELATING TO THE NURSING PROCESS

Write the step of the nursing process that is related to the nursing assistant action.

Nursing Assistant Action	Nursing Process Step
1. The nursing assistant, finding a patient on the floor, first checks the airway.	_____
2. The nursing assistant finds an unconscious patient and immediately signals for help.	_____
3. The patient stumbles, injuring her knee, which begins to bleed. The nursing assistant applies direct pressure on the wound with his gloved hand.	_____
4. The nursing assistant encourages the patient to rest quietly after a seizure.	_____
5. After summoning help for the heart attack victim, the nursing assistant remains with the patient to offer emotional support.	_____

Student Performance Record

STUDENT PERFORMANCE RECORD

Your teacher will evaluate each procedure you learn and perform, but it will be helpful if you also keep a record so that you know which experiences you still must master.

PROCEDURE	Date	Satisfactory	Unsatisfactory
Unit 13 Infection Control			
Procedure 1 Handwashing			
Procedure 2 Putting on a Mask			
Procedure 3 Putting on a Gown			
Procedure 4 Putting on Gloves			
Procedure 5 Removing Contaminated Gloves			
Procedure 6 Removing Contaminated Gloves, Eye Protection, Gown, and Mask			
Procedure 7 Transferring Nondisposable Equipment Outside of the Isolation Unit			
Procedure 8 Specimen Collection from a Patient in an Isolation Unit			
Procedure 9 Transporting a Patient to and from the Isolation Unit			
Unit 15 Patient Safety and Positioning			
Procedure 10 Turning the Patient Toward You			
Procedure 11 Turning the Patient Away from You			
Procedure 12 Moving a Patient to the Head of the Bed			
Procedure 13 Logrolling the Patient			
Unit 16 The Patient's Mobility: Transfer Skills			
Procedure 14 Applying a Transfer Belt			
Procedure 15 Transferring the Patient from Bed to Chair or Wheelchair and Back—One Assistant			
Procedure 16 Transferring the Patient from Bed to Chair or Wheelchair and Back—Two Assistants			
Procedure 17 Sliding-Board Transfer from Bed to Wheelchair			
Procedure 18 Independent Transfer, Standby Assist			

PROCEDURE	Date	Satisfactory	Unsatisfactory
Procedure 19 Transferring the Patient from Bed to Stretcher			
Procedure 20 Transferring the Patient with a Mechanical Lift			
Procedure 21 Transferring the Patient onto and off the Toilet			
Unit 17 The Patient's Mobility: Ambulation			
Procedure 22 Assisting the Patient to Walk with a Cane and Two-Point Gait			
Procedure 23 Assisting the Patient to Walk with a Walker and Three-Point Gait			
Procedure 24 Assisting the Falling Patient			
Unit 18 Body Temperature			
Procedure 25 Measuring an Oral Temperature			
Procedure 26 Measuring a Rectal Temperature			
Procedure 27 Measuring an Axillary Temperature			
Procedure 28 Measuring a Tympanic Temperature			
Procedure 29 Measuring a Temporal Artery Temperature			
Unit 19 Pulse and Respiration			
Procedure 30 Counting the Radial Pulse			
Procedure 31 Counting the Apical-Radial Pulse			
Procedure 32 Counting Respirations			
Unit 20 Blood Pressure			
Procedure 33 Taking Blood Pressure			
Procedure 34 Taking Blood Pressure with an Electronic Blood Pressure Apparatus			
Unit 21 Measuring Height and Weight			
Procedure 35 Measuring Weight and Height			
Unit 22 Admission, Transfer, and Discharge			
Procedure 36 Admitting the Patient			

PROCEDURE	Date	Satisfactory	Unsatisfactory
Procedure 37 Transferring the Patient			
Procedure 38 Discharging the Patient			
Unit 23 Bedmaking			
Procedure 39 Making a Closed Bed			
Procedure 40 Opening the Closed Bed			
Procedure 41 Making an Occupied Bed			
Procedure 42 Making the Surgical Bed			
Unit 24 Patient Bathing			
Procedure 43 Assisting with the Tub Bath or Shower			
Procedure 44 Bed Bath or Waterless Bed Bath (Bag Bath)			
Procedure 45 Changing the Patient's Gown			
Procedure 46 Partial Bath			
Procedure 47 Female Perineal Care			
Procedure 48 Male Perineal Care			
Procedure 49 Hand and Fingernail Care			
Procedure 50 Bed Shampoo			
Procedure 51 Dressing and Undressing the Patient			
Unit 25 General Comfort Measures			
Procedure 52 Assisting the Patient to Floss and Brush Teeth			
Procedure 53 Providing Mouth Care for an Unresponsive Patient			
Procedure 54 Caring for Dentures			
Procedure 55 Backrub			
Procedure 56 Shaving a Male Patient			
Procedure 57 Daily Hair Care			
Unit 26 Urinary Elimination			
Procedure 58 Assisting with the Bedpan			

PROCEDURE	Date	Satisfactory	Unsatisfactory
Procedure 59 Assisting with the Urinal			
Procedure 60 Assisting with Use of the Bedside Commode			
Procedure 61 Collecting a Routine Urine Specimen			
Procedure 62 Collecting a Clean-Catch Urine Specimen			
Procedure 63 Collecting a 24-Hour Urine Specimen			
Procedure 64 Collecting a Urine Specimen from an Infant			
Procedure 65 Giving Indwelling Catheter Care			
Procedure 66 Emptying a Urinary Drainage Unit			
Procedure 67 Collecting a Urine Specimen through a Drainage Port			
Procedure 68 Disconnecting the Urinary Catheter			
Procedure 69 Applying a Condom for Urinary Drainage			
Procedure 70 Connecting a Catheter to a Leg Bag			
Procedure 71 Emptying a Leg Bag			
Unit 27 Gastrointestinal Elimination			
Procedure 72 Collecting a Stool Specimen			
Procedure 73 Testing Stool for Occult Blood			
Procedure 74 Giving a Soap-Solution Enema			
Procedure 75 Giving a Commercially Prepared Enema			
Procedure 76 Inserting a Rectal Suppository			
Procedure 77 Giving Routine Stoma Care (Colostomy)			
Unit 28 Nutritional Needs and Diet Modifications			
Procedure 78 Serving Meal Trays			
Procedure 79 Feeding the Dependent Patient			
Unit 29 Caring for the Perioperative Patient			
Procedure 80 Assisting the Patient to Deep Breathe and Cough			

PROCEDURE	Date	Satisfactory	Unsatisfactory
Procedure 81 Performing Postoperative Leg Exercises			
Procedure 82 Applying Elasticized Stocking			
Procedure 83 Applying Sequential Compression Hosiery			
Procedure 84 Assisting the Patient to Dangle			
Unit 33 Caring for the Patient Who Is Dying			
Procedure 85 Giving Postmortem Care			
Unit 35 Caring for Patients with Disorders of the Integumentary System			
Procedure 86 Changing a Clean Dressing			
Unit 36 Caring for Patients with Cardiopulmonary Disorders			
Procedure 87 Checking Capillary Refill			
Procedure 88 Using a Pulse Oximeter			
Procedure 89 Collecting a Sputum Specimen			
Unit 37 Caring for Patients with Disorders of the Musculoskeletal and Nervous Systems			
Procedure 90 Assisting with Continuous Passive Motion			
Procedure 91 Performing Range-of-Motion Exercises (Passive)			
Unit 38 Caring for Patients with Disorders of the Sensory Organs			
Procedure 92 Caring for the Eye Socket and Artificial Eye			
Procedure 93 Applying Warm or Cool Eye Compresses			
Unit 39 Caring for Patients with Disorders of the Endocrine and Reproductive Systems			
Procedure 94 Obtaining a Fingerstick Blood Sugar			
Procedure 95 Giving a Nonsterile Vaginal Douche			
Unit 40 Caring for Obstetrical Patients and Neonates			
Procedure 96 Changing a Diaper			
Procedure 97 Weighing an Infant			
Procedure 98 Measuring an Infant			

PROCEDURE	Date	Satisfactory	Unsatisfactory
Procedure 99 Bathing an Infant			
Procedure 100 Changing Crib Linens			
Procedure 101 Changing Crib Linens (Infant in Crib)			
Procedure 102 Measuring an Infant's Temperature			
Procedure 103 Determining an Infant's Heart Rate (Pulse)			
Procedure 104 Counting an Infant's Respiratory Rate			
Procedure 105 Bottle-Feeding an Infant			
Procedure 106 Burping an Infant			
Unit 42 Response to Basic Emergencies			
Procedure 107 Head-Tilt, Chin-Lift Maneuver			
Procedure 108 Jaw-Thrust Maneuver			
Procedure 109 Mask-to-Mouth Ventilation			
Procedure 110 Positioning the Patient in the Recovery Position			
Procedure 111 Heimlich Maneuver—Abdominal Thrusts			
Procedure 112 Assisting the Adult Who Has an Obstructed Airway and Becomes Unconscious			
Procedure 113 Obstructed Airway: Infant			
Procedure 114 Assisting a Child Who Has a Foreign Body Airway Obstruction			

PART 3

Nursing Assistant Written State Test Overview

VOCABULARY

alternatives

comfort

communicate

critical points

direct care activities

distractors

handwashing

infection control

National Nurse Aide Assessment Program

patient rights

safety

skills examination

standardized test

stem

STANDARDIZED TESTING

The state certification test you will be taking is a **standardized test**. This means it was written so that it will be fair to everyone who takes the test. A test becomes standardized only after having been piloted, used, revised, and used again until it shows consistent results. The purpose of a standardized test is to establish an average score, or *norm*. This allows the results of one person's scores to be compared to the scores of many others across the state or country. A standardized test must be given in the same way each time. This is done by using the same plan and the same directions. The examiner is allowed to give only certain kinds of help. The conditions at all test sites should be similar, and each answer is scored according to definite rules.

The written state test is designed to ensure that you have the knowledge necessary to function safely as an entry-level (beginning) nursing assistant. The test varies in each state. For most states, the test has between 50 and 120 questions. You will be given approximately 2 to 4 hours to complete the written test, depending on length. Some states include approximately 10 extra questions that are not scored. These are in the process of being standardized for use in future tests. You will not know which questions are scored and which are the unscored questions. The time allowed for completing the test is fairly generous. The test examiner will call time near the end of the test to warn you that the end of the allotted time is near.

The written test questions are all in multiple-choice format. Although some questions are difficult, there are no trick questions. Questions are developed by experienced nursing assistant educators and are designed to measure the competency of an average learner. They are not designed to penalize slow learners or reward faster learners. Various terms may be used to describe the person giving care. For testing purposes, the term *nurse aide* is commonly used to describe the caregiver, but other terms, such as *nurse assistant* and *nursing assistant,* may be used in your state. The word *client* is commonly used to describe the individual receiving care, but the terms *patient* and *resident* may also be used. Your examiner will inform you of the proper terms for these individuals. The questions on the test will be placed randomly and will not be grouped together by specific category or subject.

Many states have a practice test and candidate handbook available. Ask your instructor if these tools are available in your state. They will be extremely valuable in preparing for your state test. Many practice state tests are online at http://www.promissor.com/, http://www.respondus.com/, and http://www.prometric.com/. Some state nursing assistant registries also maintain Web sites. If your state registry is online, you may wish to check its Web site for information about the state test.

STATE TEST CONTENT

The **National Nurse Aide Assessment Program** (NNAAP) forms the basis for the examination questions. The purpose of the NNAAP Written (or Oral) Examination is to make sure that you understand the responsibilities and can safely perform the job duties of an entry-level nursing assistant. The OBRA law of 1987 was designed to improve the quality of care in long-term care facilities and to establish training and examination standards for nursing assistants. Each state is responsible for following the terms of this federal law. The examination is a measure of knowledge, skills, and abilities related to nursing assisting. There are two parts to the examination: written and skills. Both parts are usually given on the same day.

The nursing assistant state written test covers the main content areas that you studied in class. These are:

Physical Care Skills

- Activities of daily living (ADLs)/Promotion of health and safety

  - hygiene

  - dressing and grooming

  - nutrition and hydration

  - elimination

  - comfort, rest, and sleep

Basic Nursing Skills

- Infection control

- Safety and emergency procedures

- Therapeutic and technical procedures, such as bedmaking, specimen collection, measurement of height and weight, and use of restraints

- Observation, reporting, and data collection

Restorative Nursing Care Skills/Promotion of Function and Health

- Preventive health care, such as prevention of contractures and pressure ulcers

- Promotion of client self-care and independence

Psychosocial Care Skills/Specialized Care

- Emotional and mental health needs

  - behavior management

  - needs of the dying client

  - sexuality needs

  - cultural and spiritual needs

Role and Responsibilities of the Nursing Assistant

- Communication

  - verbal communication

  - nonverbal communication

  - listening

  - clients with special communication problems

- Resident rights (long-term care)

- Legal and ethical behavior

- Responsibilities as a member of the health care team

- Knowledge of medical terminology and abbreviations

TAKING A MULTIPLE-CHOICE TEST

Most standardized tests use multiple-choice items. This is because multiple-choice items can measure a variety of learning outcomes, from simple to complex. They also provide the most consistent results. Each multiple-choice item consists of a **stem**, which presents a problem situation, and four possible choices called **alternatives**.

The alternatives include the correct answer and several wrong answers called **distractors**. The stem may be a question or incomplete statement, as shown in the examples.

Question form:

Q. Which of the following people is responsible for taking care of a client?

    a. janitor

    b. administrator

    c. nursing assistant

    d. social worker

Incomplete Statement form:

Q. The care of a client is the responsibility of a

    a. janitor.

    b. administrator.

    c. nursing assistant.

    d. social worker.

Although worded differently, both stems present the same problem. The alternatives in the examples contain only one correct answer. All distractors are clearly incorrect.

Another type of multiple-choice item is the best-answer format. In this format, the alternatives *may be partially correct*, but one is clearly better than the others. Look at the following example:

Best-answer form:

Q. Which of the following ethical behaviors is the MOST important?

    a. Maintain a positive attitude.

    b. Act as a responsible employee.

    c. Be courteous to visitors.

    d. Promote quality of life for each client.

Other variations of the best answer form may ask you, "What is the first thing to do," what is the "most helpful action," what is the "best response" or "best answer," or a similar kind of question. Whether the correct-answer form or best-answer form is used depends on the information given.

Each multiple-choice question lists four answers. The chance of guessing correctly is only one in four, or 25%. Each test question has only one correct answer. Do not mark more than one answer per item, or the item will be marked wrong. Do not leave answers blank.

STUDY SKILLS

No matter what type of test you take, you must first master the material. Using index cards is an excellent way to do this. The *Nurse Aide Exam Review Cards CD Package* (Thomson Delmar Learning, © 2002) is available in both English and Spanish, and is a perfect companion to your textbook. The *Nurse Aide Exam Review Cards CD Package* was designed to help ensure your success on the state test. This set of 270 flashcards will help you prepare for the state nursing assistant certification exam. Each card contains a sample question on the front and lists the question category, answer, and answer rationale on the back. Conveniently sized and completely portable, these cards are ideal for individual or group study. The cards feature questions corresponding to the National Nurse Aide Assessment Program content outline, study tips, test-day hints, and rationales with each answer. They are available as a soft-cover book, with perforated and quartered pages so you can easily remove the study cards. You may wish to prepare additional cards listing vocabulary terms, abbreviations, or questions from your workbook or text. Using index cards to create study or flashcards will enable you to test your ability to recognize and retrieve important information.

To study, read the front of the card and try to answer the question. Turn the card over to see if you are correct. After going through all the cards once, you may wish to shuffle them and review them again. Make sure you know the information and can answer questions in any order.

As you review the cards, begin to sort them into two piles. One pile is for those you know well; the other pile is those you are having trouble remembering. Once you have two piles, try to learn the most difficult information. Continue reviewing the cards until you have mastered the material. Review the cards several times a day during the time before the exam.

There are several advantages to using the card system. First, sorting the cards and preparing extra cards is a good learning experience. Looking up and writing the information on a card helps you remember it. Doing this from the beginning of class will help you immensely. Second, the cards are easy and convenient to carry with you in a purse or pocket. You can study them during spare moments throughout the day. Another advantage is that you can use the cards with a friend to quiz each other.

Other Helpful Study Skills

1. Block out a specific time for study. Study your biorhythms to learn the time of day when you function at your peak level of performance.

2. Get plenty of sleep.

3. Begin studying well before the state certification test. Schedule your study sessions so that you can take a break in between. For example, studying for an hour in the morning and an hour in the evening is more effective than studying for two consecutive hours. Trying to study when you are mentally or physically tired is a waste of time.

4. Study the most difficult material when you are most alert.

5. Control your environment. Do whatever it takes to find a quiet place to study. Get up early in the morning, when everyone else is asleep, or find a quiet corner of the library.

6. Become part of a small, dedicated study group of three to five people, or find a study partner.

7. Eat a healthful diet, especially protein and complex carbohydrates.

8. Study key concepts by asking yourself, "What are four different ways this idea could be tested?"

9. Learn the rationale behind each issue. Write a brief statement of rationale on the back of each index card with the answer. This has been done for you on the *Nurse Aide Exam Review Cards*. Study all of the information included in the rationale on your study cards. Ask yourself how the information could be tested. Make sure you can apply the principles and rationale to similar situations.

10. You may also create study checklists. Identify all the material for which you are accountable. Break it down into manageably sized lists of steps, notes, and procedures for each item. For example, write down the steps of a nursing procedure. Create a separate column for supplies needed and any special information you need to know.

11. Record your notes or study questions on audiotape. You may play the tape at home or in the car when you are commuting. The CD that accompanies the *Nurse Aide Exam Review Cards* may be used when you travel, or copied onto cassette tape if you do not have a portable CD player.

12. Many excellent tools and resources for studying are available online at http://www.studygs.net/. This site has special information for nontraditional learners, such as those with attention deficit hyperactivity disorder (ADHD); visual learners; and those who study best when they "think out loud." There are also tips for studying in groups, creating flashcards, and organizing your time.

Stress and Test Anxiety

You may be surprised to learn that stress is normal. A certain amount of stress can be good. Almost everyone has some test anxiety. Studies have shown that mild stress actually improves performance by athletes, entertainers, public speakers, and test takers! "Butterflies" in the stomach, breathing faster, sweating, and other symptoms are automatic body responses to stressful situations. Stress can sharpen your attention, keep you alert, and give you greater energy. Remember, it is not the stress that is harmful, but your reaction to it. Learn and practice how to control stress. Some stress cannot be avoided, but you will know the date of this exam well in advance. Try to avoid other stressful situations immediately before the test. Prepare yourself physically and mentally.

If you feel stressed immediately before or during the exam, try a deep breathing activity recommended by stress management experts. Breathe slowly and deeply from the diaphragm. Do not move the chest and shoulders. You should feel your abdominal muscles expand when you inhale and relax when you exhale. As you breathe out, your diaphragm and rib muscles seem to relax and your body may seem to sink down into the chair. This helps promote relaxation. Sixty seconds of controlled deep breathing helps relieve stress.

Negative Thoughts

Factors that increase stress and test anxiety are negative thoughts and self-doubt. Perhaps you have thought, "I am going to fail this exam. What will my family or coworkers think if I do not pass?" You must control your reaction to this stress and stop thinking these thoughts. Instead, say to yourself, "I have done this job successfully. I know this material, and did well in class. I am going to pass this examination." View the exam as an opportunity to show what you know and can do. Positive thinking comes before positive action and positive results. Consciously stop negative thoughts and force them out by using positive ones instead.

TAKING THE TEST

To do well on a test, you should be at your best when you start. Eat a good breakfast or lunch. Try to avoid anything that will cause stress. Dress appropriately, according to exam center requirements. Candidates who are not properly attired may be denied admission.

You must be on time to take the state test. If you are late, you may not be admitted. If you miss the test, your testing fees may not be refundable, and you will lose your money. If weather conditions are unsafe, the test may be canceled and rescheduled. If you are absent because of a valid emergency, you must promptly submit proof of this emergency to the testing service (usually within 30 days). Examples of acceptable excuses are a death in the immediate family, disabling traffic accident, illness of yourself or an immediate family member, jury duty, court appearance, or military duty. A service fee may be charged if you miss the test, even if you have proof of an acceptable excuse.

Leave for the test site early enough to arrive on time. Allow a little extra time for minor delays. In some states, you may be required to arrive up to 30 minutes early to allow time for registration, processing, verification of identification, and sign-in.

Take a watch and several (two or three) number 2, sharpened black lead pencils with erasers. If your state issues an admission letter, bring it with you and present it to the examiner. Most states have a list of supplies or identification that you must bring to be admitted to the test. Most require photo identification, and some require you to produce your original social security card, or to furnish a copy of the card. Your photo identification should be a government-issued document, such as a driver's license, state identification card, or passport. The name on the photo identification should be the same as the name used to register for the test, including suffixes such as "Jr.," "III," and the like. The photo identification card must also bear your signature. Each state gives a list of acceptable identification to candidates when they register for the test. If you do not have proper photo identification, contact the testing service well in advance to make arrangements for using an alternate means of identification. Some states require two different forms of identification. Learn the requirements in advance and be prepared to meet them. In addition, some states require fingerprinting by a law enforcement agency prior to testing. It is the applicant's responsibility to see that this has been done in a timely manner, and to pay all associated fees. You may be required to bring the official (completed) fingerprint card with you at the time of testing. If you are late or fail to bring the required identification or supplies, you may not be admitted, so follow directions carefully.

You will not be permitted to bring audio or video recording devices or personal communication devices, such as pagers and cell phones, into the test site. Likewise, you may not bring children, visitors, or pets. (Service animals are not considered pets and will be admitted.) Do not bring valuables or weapons. You probably will not be permitted to bring personal items other than your keys into the exam room. Leave purses, backpacks, books, notes, and other items in the car. You will not be permitted to eat, drink, or smoke during the examination. Students who display disruptive behavior will be removed and their exam scores recorded as a failure. If necessary, the skills examiner will call law enforcement authorities to remove or manage a disruptive candidate.

When you arrive at the test site, do not let another person's last-minute questions or comments upset you. Do not talk about the test with other students, if possible. Anxiety is contagious. Follow these general rules for taking the test:

1. Choose a good spot to sit. Make sure you have enough space. Maintain good posture and do not slouch. Be comfortable but alert. Stay relaxed and confident.

2. Remind yourself that you are well prepared and are going to do well. If you become anxious, take several slow, deep breaths to relax.

3. You will be given verbal instructions and be asked to complete an information form. Pay close attention to the examiner's instructions. He or she will read the directions. The examiner may not be permitted to answer questions.

4. Take several more deep breaths and try to relax. If you become anxious during the test, close your eyes for a few seconds and practice slow, deep breathing. Remaining relaxed and positive are keys to success. Remind yourself that you have studied well and are prepared to take the test. Think positive.

5. When you receive your test booklet, review the written directions and look at any sample questions. Make sure you understand how to mark your answers. Follow directions carefully. Most state tests are scored by computer, and stray marks can cause otherwise correct answers to be marked wrong. Write only on your answer sheet. Answers written in the exam book will not be counted.

6. Work at a steady pace.

7. Take the questions at face value. Do not read anything into them. Avoid thinking "what if?" Answer the question based on the information given. Do not look for trick questions or hidden meanings. Do not add or subtract information.

8. Read the stem of the question. Think of the answer in your own words before reading the answers. Then read all of the answers given. Search for the correct alternative, then select the option that most closely matches your answer. If necessary, read the stem with each option. If you are still not sure, treat each option as a true-false question, and choose the "most true."

9. It may be helpful to cross out unnecessary words in the question. Distracting information has been crossed out in the following example:
   Q. A client ~~who~~ is HIV positive ~~understands that the nurse aide will not talk about this information outside the facility because~~ this information is:
   a. legal.
   b. confidential.
   c. negligent.
   d. cultural.

10. If you do not know the answer to a question, circle the number and move on. Come back to it later. You may remember the answer later, or may find a clue to the answer in another question. Do not waste time struggling with questions you are unsure of. This increases your stress and test anxiety. Continuing with the test is best.

11. Be alert to words such as *not* and *except* that may completely change the intent of the question. Pay close attention to words that are *italicized*, CAPITALIZED, or are within "quotation marks" or (parentheses). Words such as *first, last, most, least, best,* and *except* often hold the key to the answer. Read carefully. These words are usually very important.

12. Avoid unfamiliar choices. Information that you are unfamiliar with is probably incorrect.

13. If you do not know the answer, try to identify answers that are not correct. Cross out answers that you know or think are incorrect. If you have crossed out two answers, you have a 50% chance of guessing correctly. Other suggestions for eliminating incorrect answers are to cross out:
    a. Question options that grammatically do not fit with the stem
    b. Question options that are completely unfamiliar to you
    c. Question options that contain negative or absolute words, such as those listed in number 11 above.

Some other strategies may also be useful:

    a. Substitute a qualified term for the absolute one, such as "frequently" instead of "always." This may help you eliminate another incorrect answer.

    b. If two answers seem correct, compare them for differences, then refer to the stem to find your best answer.

    c. Use hints from questions you know to help you answer questions that you are not sure of.

14. Look at the shortest and longest of the remaining answers. The correct answer may be shorter or longer than the others.

15. There is no penalty for guessing. If you cannot figure out the answer, guessing is better than leaving a question blank.

16. Do not become upset or nervous if some individuals finish the test early and get up to leave. Some people read faster than others. Studies have shown that those who finish first do not necessarily get the best scores.

17. When you get to the end of the test, go back and complete the items you skipped.

18. Do not change your answers without a good reason. Your first answer is more likely to be correct. Change the answer if you misread or misunderstood the question, or if you are absolutely certain the first answer is wrong.

19. Before turning the test in, check it to make sure you marked every answer. Check the circles or boxes to be sure they are completely marked on the computer scoring sheet. Erase all stray marks.

MISCELLANEOUS TESTING CONCERNS

- In some states, the written test is given by computer. If you are taking a computerized test, you will be given several practice questions to make sure you know how to use the computer. Complete the practice questions. If you have difficulty using the computer, speak with the skills examiner.

- Some states administer oral examinations. Some states give examinations in languages other than English. These special examinations must be requested from your state testing agency when you register to take the test. If you think you need an oral examination or non-English version of the test, contact your instructor or state testing service for information and instructions. The oral examinations are typically furnished on a cassette tape or CD. You will listen to the tape with a headset. Typically, each question is read twice in a neutral manner. You will also be furnished with a written test booklet so you can review the printed words while listening to the tape. You will answer the question by marking the answer sheet. However, to be a nursing assistant, you must be able to read and write in English. Even if you take an oral or foreign-language examination, you will be given a series of reading comprehension questions, typically 10. You must pass this portion of the examination, showing your understanding of the English language, in order to pass the exam as a whole. The time limits for oral testing are usually the same as the time limits for the written test.

- Your state will accommodate individuals with certain disabilities during the test. Contact your state testing agency well in advance for information on requesting accommodations. You cannot wait until the day of the test to request a special accommodation.

- Your state will have a skills (manual competency) examination portion of the state certification test. You must pass both portions of the test before being entered into the nursing assistant registry. Contact your instructor or state testing agency for information.

- *Do not bring personal communication devices, such as pagers, telephones, or other electronic devices, to the test site.* Use of these items is not permitted, and you will not be allowed to take them into the test site.

Test Security

- *Do not give help to anyone or receive help from anyone during the test.* If the examiner suspects a candidate of cheating on the examination, he or she will end that candidate's test and ask the individual to leave. The score will be recorded as a failure. The examiner reports individuals who cheat on the test to the state nursing assistant registry.

- Individuals caught removing a test from the testing site may be prosecuted. Copying, displaying, or distributing a copyrighted examination is illegal.

- When you have finished testing, turn all paper materials in. You may not remove the examination booklet, notes, or papers from the room.

THE SKILLS EXAMINATION

Part of the state test is a **skills examination**. This examination is administered slightly differently in each state. Usually, a nurse who has no affiliation with your school or educational program administers the examination. You will be tested on the number of skills required by your state. Your skills will be chosen at random from the required skills list for your state. In most states, five skills are tested.

Reporting to the nurse, documenting, and doing basic calculations are parts of some skills. For example, if you weigh a patient, you must calculate the total value from the upper and lower bars of the scale correctly. If you take a rectal or axillary temperature, you must show the skills examiner that you know how to record it correctly by placing an "R" or "A" after the temperature reading. If you count the pulse or respirations for 30 seconds, you must calculate and document the full-minute value correctly. If a value is abnormal, such as a temperature of 103.6°F (R), you must recognize that the value is abnormal and report it to the nurse or proper person. (In this case, inform the skills examiner of the abnormal value and state that you would report it to the nurse. If you are taking the test on a real patient, notify the nurse promptly as soon as the exam has ended, or ask the examiner's permission to leave briefly to report.) If you empty a catheter bag or measure intake and output, you must use a graduate, measure, calculate, add, and document the total(s) correctly. This also applies to estimating meal intake and other measurements and calculations on the examination. If you are concerned about your math skills, ask your instructor if you will be permitted to use a calculator. If so, take one with you to the exam.

The passing rate for the skills component of the exam will vary with your state. Commonly, you must pass four or five skills to pass the examination. However, you do not have to complete each skill perfectly. Certain steps are designated as critical points in the skill. If you perform these correctly, you will pass the skill, even if you make a mistake. In some states, this testing is done in the skills laboratory using other students as patient volunteers. The examiner reads the student volunteer a statement and gives instructions on what is expected in playing the role of the patient. Treat the student volunteer exactly as you would a patient. Some skills, such as perineal care, may be done on a manikin. Pretend the manikin is a patient, and treat it with the same courtesy and precautions as you would use for a patient. All equipment and supplies will be available to perform the skill, but you must know what you need and gather it before beginning. Ask questions before you begin testing on the skill. Once the test begins, the nurse examiner will be unable to answer questions.

Some states do the state skills test only on residents in a nursing facility. Some states time the skills examination. For example, you may be given 35 minutes in which to complete this portion of the test. Some states require you to pass the written test first, before you will be permitted to take the skills exam. In other states, the opposite is true: You must pass the skills examination before you will be permitted to take the written test. Although foreign-language options are available for the written test, the skills examination is given only in English.

Preparing for the Skills Examination

The only way to prepare adequately for the skills examination is to practice each procedure in sequence. If you practice, the skills will become automatic. The skills that you will be tested on are randomly selected from the procedures you learned in class. If your nursing assistant class has a review day or mock skills examination before you take the test, be sure to attend. This will be very helpful to you in preparing for the skills test.

You should also review your vocabulary terms so you are familiar with the various names for the procedures. For example, the skills examiner may direct you to "ambulate the patient." From your review of the vocabulary, you know that *ambulate* means to *walk*. If the examiner instructs you to do range-of-motion exercises on the lower *extremities,* you must know that these are the *legs*. Practice your skills with other students or with your family, and use your procedure checklists or forms provided by your state.

When reviewing the procedures, pay close attention to the list of supplies and equipment you will need to gather before you perform the procedure. It is essential that you collect the right supplies at the time of the skills test, or you may be unable to complete a procedure.

There is no way to study for the skills examination other than reviewing and practicing the procedures you learned in class. The skills examiner will watch for many things during the examination. Some of these observations are very important and may be the deciding factor in whether you pass or fail a particular skill on the examination.

Observations Made During the Skills Examination

Gather all the supplies you will need before beginning each section of the test. If you will be making the bed, stack the linen in order of use. The test will go more smoothly if you are well organized.

Direct Care

Most of the skills examination consists of **direct care activities**. Direct patient care activities assist patients in meeting basic human needs, such as feeding, drinking, positioning, ambulating, grooming, toileting, and dressing. The procedures may involve collecting, recording, and reporting information.

Indirect Care

Certain skills are part of every procedure that you perform. These are usually called **indirect care skills**. Indirect activities focus on maintaining the environment and the systems in which nursing care is delivered. They assist in providing a clean, efficient, safe, comfortable, respectful patient care environment. An indirect care skill is an important part of the procedure, but does not necessarily affect the outcome. Data collection, documentation, consultation with other health care providers, and reporting information are indirect care skills. Examples of indirect care tasks are communication, comfort, patient rights, safety, and infection control. The skills examiner will look closely at (and score) your indirect care skills in each and every procedure. Doing these things each and every time is critical to your success. Indirect care skills on which you will be tested include the following essential elements:

- The skills examiner will observe **handwashing**. He or she will monitor your handwashing technique to be sure that you follow accepted standards and procedures. Wash your hands before and after caring for each patient, and more often as necessary. This skill will not be prompted by the examiner, meaning that you will not be told or reminded to do it. Nursing assistants are expected to know when and how to wash their hands. Use the proper technique. Each handwashing should last a minimum of 15 seconds, or according to your state rules. You may be permitted to use alcohol-based hand cleaner unless your hands are soiled. Consult your instructor on this in advance. However, the skills examiner may still request you to do at least one handwash at the sink so that he or she can see whether you have mastered the skill.

- **Infection control** is another area on which you are evaluated. The skills examiner observes your technique in patient care, the use of standard precautions, and the use of medical asepsis. The examiner will also observe if you wear gloves and other PPE when necessary. You will be evaluated on whether you wash your hands before applying and removing gloves, as well as using proper technique in applying and removing the gloves themselves. Other important considerations are keeping clean and soiled items separated, disposing of soiled articles correctly, and preventing environmental contamination from used gloves and equipment.

- The examiner will observe how well you **communicate** with each patient. You must introduce yourself and the skills examiner. Explain what you are going to do, even if the patient is confused. Inform the patient before each step, such as "Now I am going to turn you over on your side." You may also be evaluated on whether you speak with the patient throughout the procedure.

- The skills examiner will observe how well you practice **safety**. In fact, many safety violations constitute automatic test failures, such as leaving the bedside with the bed in the high position and side rails down. Another example is failure to lock the wheelchair brakes before transferring the patient. These are potentially serious problems that could result in patient injuries, so the skills examiners take them very seriously. Protect patient safety throughout the procedure. When you have finished the procedure, make sure the patient is left safe, with the call signal within reach. Do not leave the room if the patient is in an unsafe location or position, or if the ordered side rails or restraints are not in place.

- Protecting and honoring **patient rights** is also very important. Be sure to knock on doors and wait for permission to enter. Use the bath blanket for modesty when the patient's body will be exposed, such as during bathing and perineal care. Pull the privacy curtain, close the window curtains, and close the door to the room. Speak with the patient in a dignified manner. Avoid terms such as "honey," "dear," "granny," and "sweetie." Although facility staff may call patients by endearing names, the skills examiner will consider it undignified and unprofessional. Treat patients with the utmost respect. The nurse examiner will monitor your attention to the patient's dignity, privacy, and safety.

- Patient **comfort** is an important consideration. You must ensure patients' comfort by doing things such as handling patients gently, asking about their comfort, supporting the arm when taking the blood pressure, positioning patients in good body alignment, and leaving each patient in a comfortable position upon completion of the skill.

Critical Points

Critical points are things that could potentially harm a patient. If you skip a critical point on your state skills examination, you will fail the skill. If your state or program uses skills checklists with key or critical points listed, pay close attention to them. For example, in many states, failure to balance the scale before weighing a patient is a critical (automatic failure) point.

Studying the critical points for each skill will be very helpful to you. Because these things could potentially harm a patient, you will feel more confident in providing care on the nursing unit. Learning the critical points for each skill creates a win-win situation for both you and the patients. The following is an example of an actual skills test from one state. The underlined steps are the critical skills or automatic failure points.

Handwashing

1. Turns on water.

2. Wets hands.

3. Applies skin cleanser or soap to hands.

4. <u>Rubs hands together for at least 15 seconds in a circular motion.</u>

5. <u>Washes all surfaces of the hands at least up to the wrist.</u>

6. Rinses hands thoroughly from wrist to fingertips; cleans under fingernails, if needed, fingers down, under running water.

7. Dries hands on clean towel/warm air dryer.

8. Turns off faucet with towel and/or <u>avoids contact with sink or other dirty surfaces during rinsing and drying of the hands.</u>

9. Discards wet towel appropriately.

When taking the skills test, think through each task that is asked of you. If the nurse examiner tells you that your patient has had a stroke with right-side paralysis, and then instructs you to get the patient out of bed, think about which side the patient will transfer to, where you will position the wheelchair, how you will keep the patient safe, and whether another assistant is needed to help. Critical points for this skill will include locking the wheelchair brakes and using a transfer belt (unless contraindicated).

Other Mistakes

If you think you have made a mistake or forget to do something during the skills examination, inform the skills examiner immediately. He or she may allow you to go back and correct the problem. This depends on the nature of the error and when you notify the examiner. If you inform the examiner of the error in a timely manner, he or she may permit you to go back and begin again at the point where the error was made. The skills examiner will not correct you if you make an error. He or she will not answer questions about the procedure during the test. If you have questions, ask them before testing begins. The skills examiner will not assist you or intervene during the test unless an unsafe patient condition develops.

AFTER THE TEST

After the test, you will breathe a sigh of relief. Listen carefully to the examiner's instructions for returning test materials. Information may also be provided about how and when you will find out the test results. In many states, you get preliminary results the same day. You will not be given a percentage or letter grade. Preliminary scores are listed as either "pass" or "fail." The results are considered preliminary until they are validated by the testing agency in its offices. After the tests are validated, you will be given a more complete explanation of your score. You should receive a report in the mail in approximately 2 weeks. If you have not received the results within 30 days, contact the examination service.

If you have passed the written and skills examinations, your name will be entered into your state nursing assistant registry. This may take several weeks. In some states, the criminal background and fingerprint checks must also be cleared before you are entered into the registry. You will be issued a wallet card to show as proof of your certification. Protect your wallet card and do not lose it. Never give your employer or a prospective employer the original. If someone needs a copy, make a photocopy and keep the original in a safe place. If you lose your card, your state will issue a duplicate, but there is usually a fee for this service. Your certification must be current for the state to issue a duplicate card. Do not alter your card in any way. Altering the card may result in loss of certification.

If you did not pass the test, you will have at least two more opportunities to retest. You have three opportunities to pass each part of the examination. However, there is a fee for each retesting. Your instructor must register you for the retest. All testing fees must be submitted to the testing service at the time of registration. Meet with your instructor to find out what to study to increase your chances of successfully passing the retest.

You must keep your state nursing assistant registry informed of any changes in your name or address. If you move or change your name, notify the state registry promptly in writing. Provide your state registration number or social security number so the information can be listed for the proper person. (More than one person may have the same name.) Many states have forms for change of name or address available on their Web sites.

Your nursing assistant certification will expire in 24 months. To renew it, you must meet your state continuing education requirements. To remain active, you must submit a form verifying that you have provided nursing assistant services for pay during the renewal period. The number of hours you are required to work to maintain your certification varies with each state.

Flashcards

abdomin/o	cephal/o
aden/o	cerebr/o
adren/o	chol/e
angi/o	chondr/o
arteri/o	col/o
arthr/o	cost/o
bronch/o	crani/o
card, cardi/o	cyst/o

head	abdomen
brain	gland
bile	adrenal gland
cartilage	vessel
colon, large intestine	artery
rib	joint
skull	bronchus, bronchi
bladder, cyst	heart

cyt/o	gloss/o
dent/o	hem, hema
derma	hemo, hemat
encephal/o	hepat/o
enter/o	hyster/o
erythr/o	ile/o
gastr/o	lapar/o
geront/o	laryng/o

tongue	cell
blood	tooth
blood	skin
liver	brain
uterus	small intestine
ileum	red
abdomen, loin, flank	stomach
larynx	old age

mamm/o	oophor/o
mast/o	ophthalm/o
men/o	oste/o
my/o	ot/o
myel/o	pharyng/o
nephr/o	phleb/o
neur/o	pneum/o
ocul/o	proct/o

ovary	breast
eye	breast
bone	menstruation
ear	muscle
pharynx	spinal cord, bone marrow
vein	kidney
lung, air, gas	nerve
rectum	eye

psych/o	thorac/o
pulm/o	thym/o
rect/o	thyr/o
rhin/o	trache/o
salping/o	ur/o
splen/o	urethr/o
stern/o	urin/o
stomat/o	uter/o

chest	mind
thymus	lung
thyroid	rectum
trachea	nose
urine, urinary tract, urination	auditory (eustachian) tube, uterine (fallopian) tube
urethra	spleen
urine	sternum
uterus	mouth

ven/o	thromb/o
fibr/o	tox/o, toxic/o
glyc/o	a—
gynec/o	ante—
hydr/o	anti—
lith/o	bio—
ped/o	brady—
py/o	contra—

clot	vein
poison	fiber
without	sugar
before	woman
against, counteracting	water
life	stone
slow	child
against, opposed	pus

dys—	poly—
hyper—	pre—
hypo—	pseudo—
inter—	tachy—
intra—	—centesis
neo—	—genic
pan—	—gram
peri—	—logy

many	pain or difficulty
before	above, excessive
false	low, deficient
fast	between
puncture or aspiration of	within
producing, causing	new
record	all
study of	around

—lysis	—rrhagia
—megaly	—rrhea
—otomy	—scope
—pathy	—scopy
—penia	—stasis
—plegia	
—pnea	
—ptosis	

excessive flow	destruction
profuse flow, discharge	enlargement
examination instrument	incision
examination using a scope	disease
maintaining a constant level	lack, deficiency
	paralysis
	breathing, respiration
	falling, sagging, dropping down